BEASTMODE CALISTHENICS

A Simple and Effective Guide to Get Ripped with Bodyweight Training

DAILY JAY

CONTENTS

Before You Start Reading!	v
Introduction	vii
Chapter One: Starting Your Journey	1
Chapter Two: Months 1-3	13
Chapter Three: Months 4-6	31
Chapter Four: The First 30 Days	39
Chapter Five: Diet and Avoiding Pitfalls	50
Chapter Six: The Ultimate Calisthenics Workout	63
Chapter Seven: When Problems Arise	91
Chapter Eight: The Cool Down	101
Final Words	103
Acknowledgments	105

© Copyright 2019 - All rights reserved.

It is not legal to reproduce, duplicate, or transmit any part of this document in either electronic means or in printed format. Recording of this publication is strictly prohibited and any storage of this document is not allowed unless with written permission from the publisher except for the use of brief quotations in a book review.

BEFORE YOU START READING!

I have this special bonus that I am going to reveal to you.

https://bit.ly/DailyJayyy

Up there is a link that will direct you to website where you can get a fitness calculator. I actually used this exact same calculator to get an estimate and track how many calories I need to eat in a day to achieve the body of my dreams when I was just getting started in my journey.

Just insert your Name and Email and the app will be sent straight to your email.

INTRODUCTION

Earlier this week, I was speaking with a friend of mine about our respective workout habits. This is a subject we had discussed many times before, but today I decided to ask a very specific question.

"Why did you start doing calisthenics?"

In our previous conversations we had talked about increasing flexibility, variations in squat positions, and appropriate set repetitions; and yet I had never asked that simple, fundamental question. Even though working out had created a great deal of positive change in my life, somehow I had overlooked that inquiry.

Despite the amount of experience I had in this particular area, my friend's purpose for it had slipped my mind. It was a question I had been asked many times when starting with a new trainer. However, it had somehow gone overlooked in my personal life. His response proved that it was a much bigger subject than I once thought.

"Six months ago, I didn't want to live anymore." Honestly, I expected to hear something similar to the other reasons I had heard over the years—increasing strength, becoming more attractive, or a variety of more surface-level issues. This was something much deeper. It was something that even I, who placed so much value and weight in working out, had not seen. I put so much of myself into working out, but all of it had been from *my* perspective and not trying to see through the eyes of others. By listening and expanding my thought process, I was able to learn so much more about a subject I considered myself fully learned in.

My friend explained that he had been experiencing a very low point in his life for several reasons, ranging from family to work. He tried to use his usual methods of coping but it merely put off the problem without repairing or bettering a thing. One day, he walked into a fitness center, took the time to sit down with a trainer, and began what he so poignantly referred to as his *journey*—the journey of calisthenics.

Maybe you aren't struggling with life in the ways my friend was, but you are reading this book to find a solution to some issue within yourself. It could be something simple and short-term, or perhaps it is a life change that will take a true journey to accomplish; either way, you are looking to calisthenics as a catalyst and guide to that change.

Or perhaps you are like myself and were unaware of how deep this lifestyle can become. It isn't easy, of course, but the changes are lasting and the scope of life-altering moments are for the better. You may have stumbled into this simply looking for your usual, small-thought workouts. Those are more of a one-dimensional approach to life's issues; a single solution for a single issue solved through one action alone. For certain personality types, or for a smaller impact, those routines work just fine. For a true change in your life, for better health and a broader mind, and for more trust in and with yourself; for all this, you need a workout that is different.

Together, we will learn new and better habits, in both your life and your workout routine. Through these proven steps, you will establish a solid baseline and discover how to build upon it for an altered, healthier life. There are likely some areas in your life that got the spotlight, as you have been reading. It is very common and can be extremely helpful to recognize this early on. Your mind and body are aware of what is needed for true repair of self, but people rarely take the time to listen hard enough. This may seem like an attack, but it is simply an observation. Because the majority of workout programs I have experienced or studied seemed to lack a multi-subject approach—as well as giving proper focus to the honesty within yourself—something jumps out when you feel heard. You may not have considered these parts of your life to need improvement, but noticing patterns that can be changed for the better is not a bad thing! It is the first part of understanding the necessary steps to alter your life for the better!

I believe it is always best to set out from a place of positivity; so let's celebrate the beginning and the journey that is about to start!

CHAPTER ONE: STARTING YOUR JOURNEY

There are many reasons why people would choose this book; and they are often very personal, as you may already know. What I mean by that is there are arcs of thought that tend to cover most workouts—devote time, work out, get better. There is too much focus on a singular area for the routine to give attention to every part that needs bettering. You had reasons before you opened the book, and I am sure you have even more by now.

As you make your way through the steps and workouts, taking the time to appreciate the achievements along the way, you will discover and fulfill your promise to yourself. It is important that there be no judgement at any point throughout this process. It will be difficult at first, but you need to be able to recognize your problem areas without allowing the degrading power (that part of you that is much too hard on yourself) to emerge. By removing judgement from the equation, you don't waste time being down on yourself and can instead focus on the solutions! Every *journey* has ups and downs, but they do not take away from both the results and the willpower gained by following through.

You've probably been here before and you may feel a bit of déjà vu. The positivity, the layout, even the wording may already have you on edge. For most people, there is a long list of workout routines that never panned out, and that is nothing to get down on yourself about! You are probably feeling that same skepticism starting up again.

Breathe. Now breathe again. One more time. Three breaths —good, solid breaths—create an excellent reset point.

Your doubt is real and should be recognized, because the promises that other programs offered you in the past fell short. Now, there will be many, many times throughout this program when you will be asked to be very honest with yourself. This may not be something you are used to, nor are comfortable with. That is also understandable. This, however, is a give and take between the reader and the program. A true relationship is one cultivated in trust and faith for the things to come; this should operate no differently! I have faith in you! Within you is a desire to better yourself in a way you haven't considered before. There is something to be said for comfort; but if the other programs were also from a source of comfort, it sounds like you need something new!

In order to get the most out of this experience, it is vital that both openness and honesty are present. To begin, be honest with yourself—what are your reasons? They have begun to show themselves in ways you probably weren't even expecting. There are no wrong answers to this question. You may have one main purpose for beginning this journey or several that combined to bring you to this point; the reasons do not matter, so long as they are important and personal to you!

CHAPTER ONE: STARTING YOUR JOURNEY

The most common reason, I have found, is weight loss.

This can come in many different forms and goals that range from a slight change to a complete life change. Your journey is your own and you need to be bonded with the foundational reasons behind it. If you only have a general idea, rather than a specific goal, that is perfectly fine! You will have plenty of time and will be given plenty of tools to identify and implement the changes you want to bring about. Consider from what angle you want to attack this weight loss; muscle endurance, mass, strength, or simple toning? By developing a strategy, you will be prepared once the action is needed.

For most people who choose this approach, they have most likely tried to attack the problem from only one angle, or the life changes weren't customized for them. That is where you will see the differences here! A multi-aspect approach to a common problem will give you the tools to not only complete and maintain the program, but to carry more confidence and ability onward throughout your life! The desired results may vary, but the drive remains the same. Even though this is common, it is unique to you and that cannot be forgotten!

There will be variations that work a wide range of muscle groups and offer different scales of impact. This will enable you to personalize the experience even more! There are alterations to focus on muscle mass and others for endurance. If you have a specific problem area you want to improve, each workout will explain the muscle groups they target. Every portion is designed to ensure that *your* journey is the best for *your* life.

Perhaps, rather than weight loss, you simply cannot find the time in your schedule to properly devote to a workout regiment. As we will touch on consistently, life does not come to a halt when a new event occurs. This program functions as an incorporation into your life rather than something piled on top of it. You'll find a better system for scheduling, a way to track the details of problem areas, and the power to overcome disruptions to that schedule. Your time is precious and important; your commitments should be as well.

Many times the scheduling isn't your issue, but rather finding a space in which to do the actual working out becomes the problem. This is no small issue, as many people continuously put off beginning a routine—or maintaining one—due to a lack of space. Having the right environment to nurture that motivation is a key tool to fighting off those distractions. Think on this as we move forward—what kind of space do *you* want? You are aware of the past attempts and where they fell short, so avoid the same missteps you made then. Don't try to make a space that you think you *should* want, and instead make one you actually *do* want. Never underestimate the impact of a safe, nurturing workout space.

All of these reasons are legitimate and, up to this point, have been stumbling blocks along the way. At no point should you feel judged. Every point brought up is designed to relate to issues you and many others have had, and still have. The important thing to remember is that no problem will be introduced or brought up without a solution being offered. You deserve to better your life and all the past reasons for not following through are going to be directly addressed and repaired!

Once you have done some inward searching, we must establish what factors led you here. By creating bonds between this experience and your personal reasons, you can build a strong foundation for the coming months. Let's break down how we can attack these "speed bumps" and turn them into motivation!

By facing these "speed bumps" head-on, you begin the process of giving the power back to yourself. Every time these "bumps" derailed a promising series of workouts or somehow lessened your drive, the power was given away. At the time, it probably did not seem as dire as I make it out to be; but the compilation of these excuses, regardless of their legitimacy, built up these "bumps" until they seemed insurmountable. Over time the mere idea of starting that regiment, because of that build-up, brings anxiety or an overwhelming feeling. In my experience, most workouts do not address these issues and instead plow forward haphazardly. This undoubtedly leads to more failures than successes and can put a bad taste in your mouth for future endeavors.

You may have noticed that a consistent tool offered in these regiments is the idea of taking time to review, preview, and list different variables. It is important that these are taken for what they are: chances to slow the speed and really get a chance to analyze. Make a conscious effort to not skip over these opportunities. Allow yourself that time to think over a situation; it could make all the difference.

Rather than using the tried-and-failed routines, together we can create an environment that renews your drive, pushes you positively towards the set goals, and finally helps you achieve the kind of lifestyle that has evaded you in the past. Remember that honesty is paramount in this journey in order to get the most out of the regiment. By attacking the root of these issues, you are empowered to push through when the days are tough. Life does not stop because you made this commitment. In fact, there will be times when life itself is enough to derail this effort. Do not be discouraged; you are more ready for this than you realize!

Let's stay in that place of positivity and take a deeper look at the life choices, or "speed bumps", that brought about this desire for change. Rather than thinking from a negative viewpoint about those reasons, let's celebrate the want to better yourself and, in turn, those around you.

Weight Loss

This is the most common reason for beginning a workout routine, although I have found it is not enough to simply want to lose weight. Usually when that is the specific purpose and goal, the problem is not a new one. Most likely, it is one that has caused you to begin many times but not truly follow through. Now look at that desire with positivity and see it for what it truly is—a selfless decision that will bring about a chain reaction of betterment in your life. This is not a singular action you are undertaking; rather, it is a series of good choices followed by even more of the same. Every single act will bring progress, and being able to fully embrace that will strengthen your base for those difficult times. Celebrate your choice here and now!

Lack Of Time/Scheduling

As I said before, life will not come to a stop when you begin this process. It is very important for you to fully understand that you are adding something to what is most likely an already busy life. That brings with it some challenges from the get-go; so start combatting those challenges with facts and logic. The best weapon is that this routine will only take 30-45 minutes from your day. If you just rolled your eyes, that is to be expected. There isn't a workout that exists without that lofty, quick-fix promise. Rather than simply throwing flashy times out there, let's take a look at what 30-45 minutes entails.

This program is time-sensitive because your time is worthwhile. Most days begin with light running—either in place or your best option—which takes around 5 minutes. From there you will go into four different exercises of varying muscle groups. Each one takes around 5 minutes as well. Only taking into account the *actual* physical actions, you've used 25 minutes. In between, it is crucial to give your body rest periods to hydrate and control your breathing; these normally take between 1-3 minutes, depending on the exercise intensity. By allowing yourself those moments, you have been working out for approximately 35 minutes. Every person is different, so there is room for extra time if needed, but that is a usual session.

When you break it down like that, it seems much more doable! Details can make a big difference as well as perspective. By focusing on the progress and actual actions, you can see exactly where your valuable time is going. In Chapter 6, we will go into even more detail to allow your scheduling complete accuracy!

Rarely are there blocks of time that go unassigned when scheduling, and that is the key roadblock for you personally. By undertaking this journey, you must accept the *addition* to that schedule. By utilizing foresight and adjusting accordingly, you can avoid any major disruptions to your daily life. Most problems when dealing specifically with time management arise because these realities were not fully understood. It is going to take some shifting and flexibility from you at the beginning in order to allow the workout it's full efficiency. You are most definitely up for this challenge! Scheduling is your strength—just look at your busy life and how you handle the day-to-day difficulties. By seeing this as a welcome addition to your life rather than an extra part that needs to fit, the positivity is sown while accepting the reality of the situation. No doubt you are already formulating times in your head, so take a breath and sketch something out. Use those gifts of time management and positively implement them now!

Finding Workout Space

I have found that this reason goes hand-in-hand with the previous one. When you cannot find the space and a gym is not an option for you, the issue of time comes into play as well. Usually, there just isn't room in the home unless it was built in or included; and if you are having trouble finding the time to work out, then the thought of any construction or redesign is daunting to say the least. This all adds up into the overwhelming feeling that tends to result in failure to follow through.

Earlier, you were asked to think about the past workout spaces you have had and how you can make better choices this time around. What were those errors? It could be something as small as not taking sound into account and discovering that your space is less noise-proof than you thought. In the past, you may have shrugged it off and pushed forward; but this time you can act with more change! You have control of this aspect and it is important for you to feel comfortable within that workout space. Everything can impact it, and the distractions should not be shrugged off; they rarely go away and usually end up returning with a vengeance later on.

Now is a good time to remember that there is no judgement

here; just like you will make that space for yourself physically, ease up on yourself mentally and emotionally. The answer lies in the simplicity of our regiment. You only need one thing to truly begin, and it has nothing to do with equipment or barbells. Your own body weight is your gym and wherever it goes, so does your ability to get that workout time in. There are varying degrees of each specific exercise which we will cover in-depth as we progress.

The important thing in this moment is to eliminate those roadblocks and excuses. Take pride in the fact that you are all you need to begin. The looming thought of investing in equipment or the fine print within a gym membership can put off even the strongest of wills; but when viewed in our positive light, it is an answer instead of a hindrance. We take small steps in the beginning to enable the sprint that will come!

There is a distinct possibility that neither of these have caused you problems in your past workouts. For some people, there is an intimidation factor in the thought of a workout program. The idea creeps in that being of a lower experience level will cause a natural halt in either motivation or ability in general. Despite previous tries, that looming sense still follows and robs you of joy and possibility in this area. For you, the key lies in adhering to the honesty within this program. Every system within this machinery was created with the intent to give accountability back to you! At the end of the day, you face yourself; so there is no better person to be your motivator on this journey! You will be empowered and built up through a natural, progressing incline. As the weeks pass, your ability will rise with it, enabling you to buy into the confidence you have been searching for.

Always remember that there is no one more capable for this than you!

These are some of the more common roadblocks that I have encountered in my experience. Yours may be different completely or a variation on what we discussed. Remember not to ignore the feelings you have during these preparedness chapters. Stay alert and confront them when they arise. Your mind and body want to have a say in this matter, and it is important to listen. Whatever brought you to this moment is a real and deep part of you that wants to change. The ability to maintain that honesty with yourself and with the steps in this book will pave the way for concrete success. Do not be deterred from your goal! If your specific roadblock was not covered, let's take some time and look inward.

The reasons behind your desire to make a change are unique and important—not just to you personally, but to the entire process. You are beginning to see the reason, or multitude of reasons, and uncovering them. Addressing them and utilizing them in a positive manner is also something you can fully achieve. The key is to not shrink away from the change you see. When a disruption rears, the natural response is to halt and worry. You will hone skills throughout this process that will enable you to focus, confront, and identify these disruptions without worry.

Depending on your past experience, the positivity that is woven into this program may be off-putting for a multitude of reasons. Whatever they may be it exists for a purpose, although it is understandable why that would be a cause for skepticism. What I have usually found is that when a program preaches a message of positivity, that is all it is built upon. Without other foundational keys, positive thinking is simply masking a form of denial.

Instead, we pair that positivity with accompanying tools that help focus that thinking into action. Rather than blindly moving forward in a bright, sunny mood, you will be instilled with real confidence. There is no rock unturned when it comes to both your physical and mental preparation, and that is where the positive thinking comes from—not a hope that things are good, but instead a knowledge that you are more than capable. From that mindset will come lasting results. That is true positivity—one that comes from a real place and is backed up with pertinent information and solutions!

Your knee-jerk reaction may be to set aside this book, but don't. Instead, use this as another chance for positivity. Discovery of self is vital—not just in this particular process, but throughout life in general. Perhaps other approaches to calisthenics haven't been as in-depth, or it is something you are not completely comfortable with. That is okay. This is not one of the "other approaches", nor will it be a comfortable journey. The design is to alter parts of yourself in such a way that habits are formed in a deep, lasting manner.

In the next chapter, you will be introduced to the program, we will go deeper into the problems you are looking to solve through this process, and we will discuss what issues with other programs led to this point as well.

The more honesty you bring to the table, the stronger your resolution will be to complete the regiment. Not only should you strive for that, but you will leave with a sense of awareness, a positive view of both yourself and the process as a whole, and, in a very real way, a life refreshed!

Chapter Summary

- How can this calisthenics workout regiment change my life?
- What brought about this desired change?
- Weight loss?
- Lifestyle change?
- Why have your past attempts not been followed through on?
- Lack of time?
- Lack of space to conduct the workout?
- Not a "gym person"?
- Honesty with yourself and the program is vital!
- Take the time to discover your personal "roadblocks".

CHAPTER TWO: MONTHS 1-3

As you begin each chapter—each forward step—it gives you a chance to reset and check that light of positivity. By now, you have given yourself permission to be honest and have discovered the reasons behind your journey. These are not surface-level variables and should be treated with respect and importance. Each step is a reminder for yourself—your reasons are real and vital to this journey. As many times as you need to hear it, repeat it one more time for luck.

Before you jump into some early looks at the physical aspect of the program, you have the chance to alter another perspective. Up to now, you have probably looked back on your past experiences quite a bit. It may be difficult at times to do this without feeling the need to be harsh. It is an understandable view—you may see your past self as someone who put you in this position and didn't follow through. More often than not, it is an overhanging sense of failure. That is a very damaging place to draw motivation from. I have rarely seen any positive results from people who work out solely from a place of avoiding failure. That perspective is incredibly effective in jumpstarting the beginning of a routine, but it burns bright, hot, and fast, leaving you burned out and more frustrated than before. This can easily become a toxic cycle of quick starts and frayed nerves.

By avoiding that label of failure, you end one cycle and begin another. Just like this program is a long-term commitment, changing a perspective—especially one with a lengthy past behind it—can prove to also be a lengthy process, but one that is incredibly worthwhile.

Now that the foundation has been laid, we can begin going into more detail regarding the actual workout. Each day along the way is another chance to take power back from those roadblocks. Just like honesty was vital in discovering your personal reasons for choosing this workout, patience is needed for every step moving forward. This is not a short event in your life; it is a vigorous, six-month routine that is designed to truly alter your life.

The more you understand the span of the program, the better prepared you will be for the marathon. You have no doubt noticed that, through repetition, you retain much more information and form habits faster. It may seem monotonous, but keep your focus on the purpose behind it. These are not just words and the exercises are not simply actions; these are methods that are all working towards a massively positive end! Your focus and effort are beginning to pay off already! Your understanding is growing and so is your appreciation for the program as a whole.

Hopefully by now you have a much wider view of your entire workout history—the times it worked, the times it didn't, and everything in-between. You will add to this more and more as you continue to learn the proper tools. In whatever method you desire, ensure that these discoveries are noted so you can refer back during this journey.

No one likes to read the instructions when they get something new; but the more time you spend on the inner workings, the better understanding you gain. The same can be said for the Ultimate Calisthenics Workout Plan. There is no lock and key preventing you from skipping ahead and simply completing the actions required. You can see some results from this method, but the truth of the matter remains—the only way to get the full impact of this process is to believe in the journey itself. As in life, without making that trek—your journey—you won't fully understand what to do with the results you gain. It seems harsh, but instant gratification rarely breeds excellence and good habits.

You know the basics and how to follow images and graphs, but when you have the backing of a deeper self, that is when the once momentary results become lasting. Rather than seeing a picture explaining the exercise, following it, and repeating, you will be able to see the workout and think back on other times you tried it as well as ways to avoid the same pitfalls this time around. You will make connections between your past self and who you are becoming now, enabling you to problem solve with a much deeper sense of change. The potential lies entirely inside you and cannot wait to begin!

Month 1

In the first month of the program, it is absolutely imperative that we lay groundwork. It may seem slow or redundant, but the actual progress you make will speak for itself. Remember, patience will be needed from the first day to the last. As with anything that requires commitment, the effort will be worth it!

Coming from a place of positivity, there has to be a focus on the environment in which you will be working out. There are many schools of thought when it comes to the actual layout of a workout area, but there is one encompassing similarity: cleanliness. Keeping a nice and tidy area is a huge step in creating the proper atmosphere for motivation! If you are of the personality type where the act of cleaning is calming, consider taking a minute at the beginning and end of each session to focus solely on cleaning. Even if that isn't something that eases anxiety, following a consistent routine in all aspects will go a long way in forming the correct habits. There is something to be said for a place where, no matter the chaos that surrounds your day and/or your physical space, peace can be found. There is control and organization that you nurture, and that is a powerful thing to have.

You will be starting with a four-day action week. This simply means that four days will be spent working out, and three days will be spent recovering. Intersperse these accordingly while making sure you try to have a rest day between action days. The start day really does not matter, although I would recommend using your usual schedule to dictate how the Ultimate Workout will be conducted. The extent to which you make these alterations are up to you. I have known people to completely scrap their usual schedule and build a new one entirely centered around their program. For the minimalist, a simple tweak here and there is all you need to allow the incorporation to occur. Keep in mind that you are not *adding* this workout program to your schedule, you are *incorporating* it. Seeing this as a priority and an organic part of your daily life will help build those foundational habits swiftly and efficiently.

In my experience, there is rarely one schedule that fits all walks of life—retail, service industry, teachers, and so on.

Even if you tend to keep a "regular" schedule—Monday through Friday, 9 AM to 5 PM—using this format still might not be the most efficient. This idea may seem daunting at first. For the most part, there is a tendency for people to stick to one main schedule and to work everything else around that. The idea of something as intensive as this workout being brought in *and* altering a schedule that has been a mainstay is intimidating, for certain. But remember, you take your power back by acknowledging the reality rather than shirking from it.

From that place of power, you can then begin the changes to your schedule. The important thing to remember is that a flexible, open mind is less prone to frustration. You will be able to see more chances for productivity if you aren't locked in to one singular method. As you make your way through the schedule, be ready to recognize any stress triggers. These can occur when you suddenly realize that you didn't include an event to the calendar and have to alter it. Don't stress over the time because you are most likely seeing it as a loss. You have lost nothing; rather, you have given yourself another opportunity to conduct the proper change. Breathe and begin the solution right away! The longer you allow that issue to remain unaddressed, the more power you grant it.

We'll break it down in a less-complex way so you can apply it to whatever schedule you may keep:

- <u>Day 1</u>: Full Body 101
- <u>Day 2</u>: Rest
- <u>Day 3</u>: Full Body 101
- <u>Day 4</u>: Rest
- <u>Day 5</u>: Full Body 101
- <u>Day 6</u>: Rest
- <u>Day 7</u>: Full Body 101

<u>Muscles worked out in Month 1</u>: Full leg muscles, glutes, abdominals, pectorals, upper arms, and shoulders

Now that you have something more concrete to consider, take a moment to plan out your first month accordingly. Be honest with yourself. Nothing is gained from overreaching, so there is no need to rush this process. You should always feel free to set this book aside and take the time to map things out. Other than your Workout Journal, keep another pad to jot down improvements or thoughts you have while reading. Some people don't mind writing directly on the page while others consider that idea quite horrific, or you may be reading this on a tablet/phone. However you keep track of these details, ensure that somehow you do. A fleeting thought mid-paragraph can easily be lost, so keep that pad handy and allow the thoughts to flow throughout the process!

Remember that the way we phrase a situation has a direct effect. This is your *journey*. This is the time to organically add this to your life. It should fit in a way that is easy to maintain without disruption. Don't give yourself a reason to back out by skimming over something this important.

Before we begin previewing the upcoming months and the exciting possibilities, it is imperative that you understand the importance of the rest periods between workout sets. Later on, we'll go into more detail on just how you can get the most recovery from those periods. For now, we can focus on the basics:

- Ease into the rest period. Avoid sudden stops in transition.
- Controlled breathing will help maintain your heart rate during the rest
- Avoid sitting or becoming motionless

You are going to be using a four-week format for each month of the program. For the more detail-oriented reader, don't place too much focus on the date, but rather the day of the week. This is a space you are crafting that will alleviate stress and promote motivation, so use a method that is comfortable for you! There will be many times during this program where you will feel uncomfortable and will be pushed, so find ways to keep some form of recuperation in that comfort. It could be something as simple as using an unorthodox ink color (or multiple colors) to track your workouts, or something more complex like an entire Excel worksheet dedicated to getting every detail you can. Make it your own!

The first month will be very generalized in regards to muscle focus. Each workout is considered Full Body and is vital in building the core for the future. Even though we are starting from a low-impact place, use this time to solidify how you see and contextualize your workouts. Don't let the rest days be considered a "day off". Focus instead on the rest and allow your body time to revitalize. If you are using a specialized diet along with this program, then these rest days are a chance to meal plan or fill in your workout journal, which we will discuss in detail later.

As we will go into more in Chapter 4, this is one of the more important stretches of time in the program. You will be building bonds with your foundation, learning a new routine, adjusting to whatever alterations you have made to your schedule, and balancing a new physical stress. It isn't a small undertaking, but that fact makes it all the more impressive!

Your mantra is this: patience. It is worth repeating. You will not see any real results until you hit that 30-day mark. Remind yourself of this often, because there *will* be moments during this first month where you get discouraged. You will be putting in a great deal of effort, and the feeling that nothing is changing can be the number one reason for ending a program prematurely. The more prepared you are for the reality of a long-term workout such as this, the more motivation ammunition you give yourself! Invest in this knowledge now and, as you progress, you will be at ease and fully ready to face each day and session! Focus instead on the other positive effects by asking a few honest questions.

How do you feel throughout the day?

Just like you will be documenting the changes in yourself during this program, note how you feel before. Take that moment and analyze your morning, midday, and night moods and general health. If there are other people in your household, check in with them and see what changes they have noticed. It can help to have multiple sets of eyes to catch every detail. Being able to plainly see different aspects of your life improving in front of you thanks to all your hard work can be very interesting and rewarding!

Are there better ways to rest yourself to avoid injury?

This doesn't just mean your Rest Days and resting times during a workout. Are you aware of your sleeping positions? What soreness do you experience right out of the gate in the morning? These can be clues to help avoid injury down the line. Your body is going to be tested more than it is used to, and there will be nights and following days that bring aches and groans. By taking notice of your physical habits, you can be better informed on where the adjustments need to be made!

Are you sleeping better?

After the first few days of working out, you can start to make this a focus as well. We will get more into the importance of sleep later, but for now simply notice what your sleep habits were and how they begin to change. There may be times when your sleep suffers, and you will need to address that as well. No matter the direction your sleep goes, you can ensure you will be prepared for it!

These are just a few self-check questions that can help chart your progress in more than a visual way.

Month 2

The second month of the program is going to keep the same four-day workout, three-day rest cycle as Month 1. The variations are in the form of different workouts and increased impact and repetitions. You will not see a large amount of difference from the types of exercises; however, the way you go about doing them will start to change. In this way, calisthenics are very much like mathematics—you build on what you learned before in order to accomplish the current task. By taking your time in the first four weeks, you will have given yourself that foundation to properly build upon.

Your muscle group focus is going to stay very general. Consider this a step up from the first set. If Month 1 covered Full Body 101, then we are moving to Full Body 102 for

Month 2. The exact workouts and details are further explained in Chapter 6, but we are creating that base for the moment. As before, map out the second month the same way you did the first. You should have an idea of how things will fit into your life and what pitfalls to avoid from the first month of scheduling.

- Day 1: Full Body 102
- Day 2: Rest
- Day 3: Full Body 102
- Day 4: Rest
- Day 5: Full Body 102
- Day 6: Rest
- Day 7: Full Body 102

Muscles worked out in Month 2: Full leg muscles, glutes, pectorals, abdominals, biceps, and backs

As we remember to move forward in positivity, this is another chance to celebrate a milestone! Two months of hard work and planning have gotten you to this point! With each day and workout, you are presented with a new opportunity to solidify your foundation.

As you make you way further into the program, you will have already encountered a good variety of exercises. The entire workout follows an upward incline in intensity and impact, but the difficulty will consistently remain at a steady, even pace. This is not a situation where you will ever feel left behind! During the detailed workouts further in the book, you will be given images and explanations to guide you along and make the process smooth. Frustration only leads to improper form and stilted breathing, neither of which helps to cultivate a positive atmosphere.

As we take a moment to look back on the progress thus far, a new roadblock may be forming or has already begun to take ground: boredom.

It seems odd when looking at it from the beginning, but by the time you reach this two-month, milestone there is a good chance that you have felt the twinge of monotony. No doubt there have been days that didn't pan out according to your calendar and times when you simply didn't feel like working out. Despite beginning and continuing from a place of positive thinking, there is no shame in understanding why you are feeling bored. It is a strange place, that plateau of eight weeks. You haven't reached the halfway point and the visual results may not be showing—the reasons to let that doubt creep in will begin to present themselves. This is not to be taken lightly. Remember, taking back power is a very large component of your journey. Don't shy away from facing this directly; you owe that to yourself.

When times like this arise, it is imperative that we use our tools of self-awareness. You know yourself very well, and this program has helped you discover foundational issues along the way.

Perhaps the details are overwhelming and you need to take a step back. View the program in its entirety rather than seeing every moment. By seeing it from that perspective, you can map out other times you felt distraught or less than inspired. Those were key moments, and I am sure you can recall the inner struggle that you went through to regain power. From the start, you have been asked to use your past as a tool for discovering present solutions, and this will be no different. It is a skill that is continuously sharpened, and for good reason.

With each moment you turn from a low point to a teachable one invests in your confidence—not just now, but for life continuing after. You are building a foundation that will be lasting and stronger than you had previously thought. That is well worth the effort! That same fire and fight can be put to work in any future situation as well. Reminding yourself that this isn't something new and that you overcame it before can be that spark you need to get you through.

Some people, instead, need the details to understand the purpose of the journey. Seeing the forest doesn't ignite anything, and instead brings a haze. By focusing on the individual workouts and days—seeing how you plotted your course—you can navigate your doubt. Break everything down to the core components and lay it out. You can see the magnitude of what you have already accomplished in plain text. Read back over your previous entries you made in the Workout Journal—again, we will cover this in detail later. The key is giving yourself detailed reminders, in detail of times you pushed through.

Both schools of thought will accomplish the same goal so long as they are applied correctly. Again, we revisit that core principle of honesty with yourself. You know the inspirations that got you to this point and as long as you follow that same path of honesty, you will have many more milestones to celebrate!

Month 3

The third month is where we introduce the first big change to your routine. The foundation is set, and I know all the work you have put in so far will begin paying off! Again, as we do to remind ourselves, begin this month with a fresh mind and preparedness. You have your schedule at the ready with pencil in hand—or pen, if you're feeling adventurous! You deserve a moment to recognize what you have achieved to this point. Plan out some extra time for this recognition! Like you did at the end of four weeks, this is your chance for a little applause. You have charted your progress and by making it this far you have started to feel and live better. There has been a commitment to honesty throughout this process, and that will continue now.

With twice the knowledge since you began this journey, you are beginning to see the patterns that your workouts are taking. You have a better sense of the pitfalls and times that strain you more than others. This is another chance to better yourself. Going into the third month, are there any tweaks you need to make? Is the schedule you have set still the best way to proceed? Taking the time to properly ask and subsequently answer these questions will increase your already impressive preparedness. You have put the work in, both physically and mentally. Be proud of yourself!

The third month of our program has two possible choices for you depending on where you find yourself. Again, being honest with yourself is paramount. By transparently evaluating yourself and your progress, you know best what level of intensity will fit. Don't be afraid to tinker with the schedule if needed. You may find that staying at the lower level isn't as challenging as you thought and you need to increase the impact. No problem! The same can be said for the reverse; if you find the higher intensity too much, ease up and find that level where progress is made without risk of injury. Remember, no judgement!

It is important to remember as you make this decision that there is also a system for adding intensity and impact to a routine through increased sets and repetitions. This program sees the third month as the vital launching point for the second half of the workouts. Because of this, it is the only month that gives you a guideline for a higher impact schedule. Before you commit to either one, review the other options for increasing the workout overall, as described in Chapter 7. The customization of the routines are foundational in creating an open and flexible environment.

The next step in this process is considered Intermediate 101. You will find a higher degree of difficulty while still building our foundation. The options will differ in your workout days and rest days, depending on what you decide. If you want to remain at a lower intensity and the challenges have progressed correctly thus far, you will follow the Low-Impact schedule. However, if you need added intensity and your schedule can avoid disruption, proceed to the High-Impact schedule.

The High Impact schedule will substitute a "Light Running" day for a Rest day to push you that extra bit. On the Light Running days, you should jog for 20-30 consecutive minutes, be it in place, on a treadmill, or outside in the beauty of nature. Whichever you choose, you will feel the added impact; but make sure you adhere to the *Light* aspect and make that simply a more active Rest day, if you will.

Remember that in order to honestly evaluate yourself, you have to come from a place without judgement, as you have throughout the journey. It may seem repetitive, but there is nothing more valuable to the success of this program than the accountability you build with yourself. It enables you to relate to each session on a very personal level.

- Low-Impact Schedule:
- Day 1: Intermediate 101

- Day 2: Rest
- Day 3: Intermediate 101
- Day 4: Rest
- Day 5: Intermediate 101
- Day 6: Rest
- Day 7: Intermediate 101
- High-Impact Schedule:
- Day 1: Intermediate 101
- Day 2: Rest
- Day 3: Intermediate 101
- Day 4: Light Running
- Day 5: Intermediate 101
- Day 6: Light Running
- Day 7: Rest

Muscles worked out in Month 3: Full leg muscles, glutes, pectorals, and back

WHEN YOU ARE PLANNING out your third month, you must place additional focus on your rest days. These are incredibly important to you achieving your goals, and how you schedule and utilize them has a direct impact, especially if you have chosen the High-Impact schedule.

Take the time now to review the schedules you have put together so far. You have a better understanding of what each session and cycle will entail, so you can take note of alterations that are needed. Specifically regarding Rest Days, here are a few useful tips and questions that will help you notice patterns that signify a change is needed:

- Are there any personal events that happen in the first three months that will require more rest after,

or that will have a large impact on your sleep schedule?
- Take special note of the Rest Days that follow back-to-back workouts to avoid disruptions from soreness or exhaustion.
- Are you comparing your current schedule to your previous workout attempts? Are any old patterns emerging that could derail your progress?
- If you chose the High-Impact schedule, do you need to do an honesty check to ensure that you will still have the proper recovery time?

Celebrate! You have reached the critical halfway point of this program! I am sure the going has been tough at times, but I know that a sense of pride accompanies this moment. You adapted and adjusted events in your life, and I know you are seeing these sacrifices paying off. By now, you should be feeling a multitude of effects across your life—physical, emotional, social, and so on. You implemented very important tools into your life and it is necessary to take a moment and consider how they have helped you outside of the workout space. You are crafting and nurturing a lifestyle that will have positive ripples long after the last page of this book.

The next three months will bring a variety of new exercises as well as bringing some old ones back! No matter if you are doing an exercise for the first time or the fiftieth time, your form is where all the efficiency is! By remaining self-aware, you will be more cognitive of slips in breathing or movements. You have quite the collection of useful tools that will no doubt lead to continued success long after this program has ended!

Chapter Summary

CHAPTER TWO: MONTHS 1-3

- A breakdown of the first three months of the Ultimate Calisthenics Workout
- Month 1
- How to schedule Workout Days and Rest Days
- Brief explanation of muscle focus
- Month 1 workout schedule
- What muscles are worked out this month?
- Month 2
- Full Body 101
- High and Low Impact schedules
- Light Running days
- Importance of Rest Days
- Patience!
- Month 2 workout schedule
- What muscles are worked out this month?
- Month 3
- How to combat boredom
- Intermediate 101
- Difference in Month 3 workout options
- Break down of Low Impact/High Impact schedule
- Month 3 Low Impact workout schedule
- Month 3 High Impact workout schedule
- What muscles are worked out this month?
- 3-month summary
- What to ask yourself now…
- What tools have you used to avoid skipping ahead or cutting corners?
- What day will start your Workout Schedule?
- Why that day?
- During the first 30 days…
- How do you feel throughout the day?
- Are there better ways to rest yourself to avoid injury?
- Are you sleeping better?

- What steps are you taking to combat boredom/monotony?
- Are you taking the workout changes in Month 3 into account?
- Do you need to adjust your Workout Schedule?

In the next chapter, you will be introduced to the second three-month cycle of the workout regiment. This will include simplified schedules for each four-week period.

CHAPTER THREE: MONTHS 4-6

As you begin this next part of the journey, it is important to restate that this is a celebratory moment. Just as you made it a point to recognize completing the first three months of the program, taking the time to celebrate beginning the next cycle is vital as well. Every recognition moment is a chance for you to refocus on a place of positivity —to notice when a breath and a cheer is needed.

It is no small feat, reaching this point. The time spent building a solid foundation, as you have, creates an atmosphere of growth. You have faced difficulties and you overcame them in every instance—scheduling, keeping reliable journal entries, and managing a non-stop life all the while. The next three months will not be easy; but because of the efforts you put in before now, you will certainly rise to each challenge!

Month 4

The next four-week cycle, Month 4, is a higher-impact focus

on the muscle groups. The routine returns to a simplified schedule—as shown below—but the exercises themselves are more advanced. Remember to not feel defeated or disheartened! You have earned these challenges and are more than capable of handling them!

In Chapter 6, when we get into the detailed workouts and their respective diagrams, there will be several options when executing the routines. Not only are there ways to increase the impact of an exercise, but there are ways to lessen it as well without removing sets or reps. These options are not designed to be a permanent substitute for the original routines; but in the case of struggling or pain, you will be able to lessen the strain for the moment.

The aim of this program is simplicity and user friendliness. It's just like when you operate a computer—the screen can be fancy and sleek, but unless the user can fully operate it with confidence and ease, none of that matters. Your results are not purely aesthetic and the more effort and time spent on the foundational ideals discussed, the deeper the impact.

Some of the exercises, as shown in Chapter 6, are normally executed using a bar or similar equipment. It is not necessary to complete the program and great care has been taken to replace complex gym maneuvers with easy-to-follow actions to get the best results for the session!

- Muscle Impact 101 Schedule:
- Day 1: Muscle Impact 101
- Day 2: Rest
- Day 3: Muscle Impact 101
- Day 4: Rest
- Day 5: Muscle Impact 101
- Day 6: Rest

- Day 7: Light Running

Muscles worked out in Month 4: Full leg muscles, glutes, abdominals, full arm muscles, shoulders, and back

REMEMBER when you schedule this cycle to take into account the rise in intensity. You may need to change the start day to allow for a more natural integration. By taking the time to properly chart this out now, you will eliminate one task when you reach the actual workout section. Use this formula as we move forward. Each cycle increases in difficulty and intensity, and it is necessary to schedule accordingly.

By this point, you are well-versed in mapping out the month's routines. Simply by reaching this part of the program, you have shown that your life and the Ultimate Calisthenics Workout are symbiotic. Not only have you turned a new addition to your life into a welcome habit, but I am sure you have a list of the ways you feel better. With that in mind, now is perfect to take a moment and create that very list! Celebrating your personal accomplishments are a vital part of your mental workouts, and seeing them laid out before you makes the gravity of your success all the more real! Do a quick self-check using the handy questions we provided earlier:

- How do you feel throughout the day?
- Are there better ways to rest yourself to avoid injury?
- Are you sleeping better?

In fact, this is another perfect moment to recognize you!

Take some time and allow yourself to breathe. As you do, list the changes you have noticed in your life. List the different ways you have gained more energy! How are you being more active? By speaking these out loud or writing them down, you are making an extra effort for yourself. It is something you deserve; after all, you have put in months of hard work!

With a mere two months remaining in our time together, make sure you look back as much as you look forward, as we always have. In the early part of this book, we stated that this was not a race—you are not in competition. Allow me to alter that slightly now. You are in competition, but it is only with the past version of yourself. No one else can know the true depth of the changes like you can. Utilize this self-awareness! Enable yourself to see this from two simultaneous perspectives, if you will. The first being one of eventual completion—the program is winding down and the end is in sight. The second, and just as important, is that there isn't much time left!

Now, I don't mean that in a panic-inducing way. That is contradictory to the entire purpose. Instead, use the second point of view as a chance to appreciate where you've come from and the progress along the way! It has already been quite a journey for you and there is a great deal of pride in that.

By combining these two views, you will have a much better grasp on the final two months. Just as with every cycle and statement before, make sure you see from that light of positivity. Your time is precious and the devotion you've shown is certainly something to think about.

Month 5

CHAPTER THREE: MONTHS 4-6

The fifth month, our second-to-last, begins to combine earlier sessions into newer ones to create a more customized routine. When you are actually executing these exercises, you can refer to the provided diagrams in Chapter 6 at any time.

As with Month 4, if an exercise has the option of equipment, it is not necessary to get the most out of the actions. You will always be given the best versions of the exercise even without equipment. This is to make sure your schedule and setup are best utilized.

- Muscle Impact 102 Schedule:
- Day 1: Muscle Impact 102
- Day 2: Intermediate 101
- Day 3: Rest
- Day 4: Muscle Impact 102
- Day 5: Intermediate 101
- Day 6: Rest
- Day 7: Light Running

Muscles worked out in Month 5: Full leg muscles, glutes, biceps, and back

DON'T PUT any pressure on yourself in regards to scheduling. Throughout the program, you have found the correct times and days in which to create a productive environment; and you've done it well! Apply the same focus to Muscle Impact 102. Refer back to your workout journal entries for Month 3 (Intermediate 101) and take them into account. Keep in mind that you have been judgement-free up until now, and there is no reason to halt that streak! Adjustments are perfectly fine and sometimes necessary to create that atmosphere. You are the subject and the focus! Your commitment has been followed through and I know the same will continue!

Month 6

Take a deep breath; you have reached the final month!

As you enter this state of finality—and a well-deserved one, at that—use the tools you picked up along the way to properly celebrate this milestone! From a blank slate to this moment, you have persevered! By this point, you have a full grasp of the exercises, scheduling, and everything in between. This will all be needed for the final month.

Thanks to all the knowledge you have in your possession, we can go straight into the final routine. As before, we will be combining previous routines to form a comprehensive and completed cycle. Month 6, known as The Ultimate Calisthenics Workout, will test all of the factors you have built up. You know your limits and how to properly rest and recover, so keep them in mind when you are scheduling this month. There is no need to rush through this. I know you can see the finish line, but there is more to be run yet.

- The Ultimate Calisthenics Workout:
- Day 1: Muscle Impact 101
- Day 2: Muscle Impact 102
- Day 3: Rest
- Day 4: Muscle Impact 102
- Day 5: Light Running
- Day 6: The Ultimate Calisthenics Workout
- Day 7: Rest

Muscles worked out in Month 6: Full body workout

CHAPTER THREE: MONTHS 4-6

By keeping to the schedules you make and believing in yourself, you've made it through the program! Use this chapter as a reference while you move forward. Your journey is personal and unique to you. This is quite the accomplishment!

As you continue onward, you will find the answers to common troubles that arise along the way, in-depth focus on the first 30-day period, and the full, diagramed Ultimate Calisthenics Workout. Every chapter is a new tool that will help you maintain and follow through like you were never able to before! Stick to the foundational basics and you can't go wrong: honesty, efficiency, and honesty again!

I celebrate you as this journey continues to better your life!

Chapter Summary

- Have you taken the time to celebrate getting to the halfway point?
- Month 4
- Review Muscle Impact 101
- Have you reviewed the upcoming changes in your workouts?
- As with Month 3, do you need to adjust your schedule?
- Will you be using a bar/equipment or is that not possible/preferred?
- Make sure you have the correct routines according to your preferences
- What muscles are worked out this month?
- Month 5
- Were you able to complete Month 4 without disruption? If not, how did you correct the situation?

- Do you have more energy?
- Are you more active?
- Review Muscle Impact 102
- Are you rushing your sets/reps or letting posture slip?
- Are you keeping up with your Workout Journal?
- What muscles are worked out this month?
- Month 6
- Have you celebrated reaching the final month?
- Review any problem areas you have encountered in the last 5 months
- Is your schedule prepared for the final month?
- Review The Ultimate Calisthenics Workout
- Review all diagrams associated with The Ultimate Calisthenics Workout to ensure familiarity and efficiency
- What muscles are worked out this month?

In the next chapter, we will focus specifically on the first 30 days of this process, the importance of using that time to form the correct habits with confidence, and a deeper look at the importance of a Workout Journal.

CHAPTER FOUR: THE FIRST 30 DAYS

It is a well-known piece of trivia that it takes thirty days to form a habit. This was taken into consideration as our workout routine was created. The first thirty days are crucial to any action plan, and this is no different for one as intensive as the Ultimate Calisthenics Workout. In the previous chapter, we examined the different pitfalls during this experience, but now we can go into more detail in regards to that foundational starting period.

Why is thirty days important? Not only are these the formative days that will have a direct impact on the following five months, but the most common period of time to drop a workout routine is within those first four weeks. It makes sense when you think about it—the habits haven't formed yet, the commitment is new, and to be honest, the investment is still low. The approach to this program took that fully into account as well. By the time you make that first movement in your first session, you will have made a solid investment in yourself already! You will have spent some real time learning about yourself and creating bonds and trust in the new choices you are making.

Every milestone and moment during your journey is important; but by focusing on the first cycle, it gives the chance to build a foundational habit. Taking every day as it comes and allowing yourself to absorb as much information as possible is a direct investment into yourself and the results you know will come! Every skill and tool you obtain during this time will be put to use in every following cycle. Remember, you are the focus!

It is within this time period that you will experience a higher chance for roadblocks.

Some days, the workout can feel like an intrusion on your usual schedule; that is a direct chance to alter your perspective. By taking action immediately, you are laying important groundwork! When you experience these moments, take the extra time to journal them. You know yourself the best! Utilize your workout journal in a way that is the most efficient *for you*!

As the program progresses, the focus will shift from foundational to the application of that knowledge. Without the proper time given early in the workouts, you will find more difficulty further down the road. With all of this in mind, the key to not only completing the first month, but getting the most out of it, is accountability. That is, without a doubt, imperative to your success!

You and yourself—that is who this contract is between. Some people have workout partners, gym buddies, and the like. This is a personal event for you and should be treated as such. We discussed the importance of honesty with yourself, and that ties directly into accountability. You have to be firm

CHAPTER FOUR: THE FIRST 30 DAYS

and stick to the commitments your scheduling creates. Don't overreach! You are yourself and any attempt to create a workout that doesn't fit you will result in more difficulty than is necessary.

Take some time to look over the detailed workouts for the first month in Chapter 6. Note that they are not advanced in nature. Sometimes not knowing what one is getting into can cause undue stress; so, educate yourself fully on what this beginning cycle entails. The focus should be correct form and adherence to repetitions—the glitz and glamor will come later. As you learn to use your workout journal to its fullest capacity, you can jot down notes to ensure you get the most out of each session. Imagine yourself in the middle of Month 5 and you are finding a specific position more difficult than usual. Take a moment and look back on your entries from when you were learning that position. Thanks to your efforts, you can see differences in how to correctly execute the position! No more unnecessary pain, plus you get the full impact of the workout!

Without taking the time to make that first month as comprehensive as possible, you rob yourself of knowledge in the future. If it helps, continue envisioning your future self and what would best help them through. As long as you and your betterment are the focus, you are on the right path!

Looking back can often help improve the forward progress! As we previously discussed, this is most likely not your first attempt at maintaining a workout regiment. Before you go to a place of judgement—which we never do—remember that by being able to see your past mistakes or pitfalls you will be empowering for you this time around!

Take some time and list every past attempt you remember. Try to be as detailed as you can—the more you can understand about those experiences, the more you can fix! As you go through the list, you will start to see patterns emerge that will tell a clearer story about your workout history. Is there a specific place in the routine that tends to burn you out? Maybe you found that you were trying too much too soon and caused injuries. These may be difficult questions, considering that the case study is you, but that just gives you a special perspective on the matter.

As you go through your list of workouts you may find times when you want to be less than honest with yourself. This is incredibly common. After all, it is just between you and yourself. The accountability falls solely to you.

Now, take a moment and breathe…

That was an intense statement, and it is important to take it all in. While a variety of patterns cause a slowing and eventual halting of the workout itself, there tends to be a common denominator: lack of accountability. It can take many forms—letting slips in schedules go, "there wasn't enough time", "life happened", and so forth. These are all real and viable occurrences and in no way should the impact be lessened. That being said, a workout is like any other commitment in your life—it takes time, effort, and then more time again. It is for these reasons that we spent so much time on scheduling.

Your life is important, and the activities and events that fill it are just as important. When you set out on this journey, a vital part of the preparation was to be honest about if this was something that could viably be assimilated into your daily life. Considering we find ourselves here, I can assume that you did indeed make that commitment to yourself. *This* is important to you too. If it wasn't, you wouldn't be pushing

CHAPTER FOUR: THE FIRST 30 DAYS

yourself and making life a little uncomfortable for the sake of personal growth!

You are more than capable of accomplishing all this and more! There is no doubting yourself here!

While you are using these first thirty days to perfect habits that will lead to success, it is just as important to shift some focus to the tracking throughout. Depending on your personal preferences, the idea of keeping a detailed account of your workouts can be quite daunting. It may seem like just another added pressure to an already stressful situation. If this is the case and the subject brings about anxiety, there are several ways to combat it. Remember, the pressure you feel is real and you shouldn't feel any shame from it. By admitting that it does cause an issue, you are giving yourself the chance to solve a life problem!

Maybe you've never really been the type to keep a journal of any kind. I had a friend when I was younger who tried and tried to keep a journal just like many of us did at that age. Every single time it was the same result—a new, blank book that was filled with potential! After a few entries, the well of motivation dried up, and a few months later it was simply forgotten. It may have seemed like a small thing—a quirk rather than a real issue—but it was not something my friend was willing to let go. Rather than get frustrated time and time again, he was able to step back and see the patterns he had developed. He recognized that there was a sense of motivation inside him; it just seemed to dim as he pushed at it. When he was able to be more honest with himself, he said that he was never a big fan of a physical, written journal. It was the common choice and what our friends were able to do, so he never considered a different method to accomplish the same goal. He did *want* to keep a journal; he just needed a different medium. To this day he still uses a small, handheld voice recorder to keep his audio journal; and to this day, the lesson of that situation has stuck with me.

The overall school of thought that keeping this account of your workouts is an incredibly positive factor, for the experience allows for many forms of actually doing it. There are digital versions for those who prefer a screen, there are helpful fill-in-the-blank workbooks to accompany a routine, and then there is the classic blank notebook method. The choice of which is yours and it should be one influenced by *you alone*!

To start from the beginning, why is a Workout Journal so important? Not only is that an excellent question, but it has to be one that you answer. Just as the first thirty days will build physical habits within your workouts, this practice of tracking your progress and noting any issues will solidify habits of organization! There are many unknowns when you are undertaking something like this program, but one absolute is that you will want something to reference down the road. As you read in Chapters 2 and 3, you will be building on previous knowledge as you move through the specific workouts. More often than not, in my experience, there will come a time when an issue will arise or some stumbling block that begins to disrupt a session or more. Rather than having to start without any prior information, you will have at the ready a detailed solution guide; and it's one that you've written yourself!

Now that we've established how vital the Workout Journal will be to this process, we'll break down the different elements that make up something of such importance. We'll focus on the specific details that you will be tracking and different formats that may be helpful.

While every individual has their own preferences when it comes to the actual layout, ensure that you are meticulous in these areas:

- Accurate date/times
- Current weight
- Specific exercise
- Sets
- Repetitions
- Problem/Success notes

These variables will provide a clear and efficient account that you can, and will need to, look back on during this program. Take some time and consider how you want to proceed with the actual journaling portion. When I was making my first functional Workout Journal, I looked over some old work, essays, and such to see if I had a comfortable way to document data. I also spoke with an old friend, the same one from the Introduction, to get another perspective on journaling.

Now, it is important to remember that these are simply examples of formats that worked in certain scenarios, and they may not fit your lifestyle or schedule. That is perfectly okay! If you haven't already, take some time now to at least skim over any of your old documents to get an idea of your specific patterns. The main purpose for the examples is to get you thinking outside the box a little. Once you have a general process in mind, use the next examples to expand your thinking to see if there are any areas of improvement.

When I went through my old journal attempts, I saw a pretty basic layout with a primary focus on the changes from week to week. I was consistently thorough when it came to those details and the data was impressive. Despite that, every journal ended the same way—a slow tapering off until it just stopped. Rather than turning to a place of judgement, I took a breath and used it as a glaring error in my process that I had the opportunity to repair.

I began putting a more even focus across the board, and I realized that my notes were more spread out among the data fields. Before, I simply had a block of text below the numbers that, in all honesty, became daunting. I didn't feel like reading paragraphs to find out information and I used that negativity to justify my deteriorating motivation. I wasn't being realistic or self-aware in those moments. I am a fast-paced person and I was not taking that into account. When I altered that and began jotting short, concise notes in all the data fields, it made for a quick reference guide! I had been mimicking methods that had been successful for others, but it did not translate correctly to myself. Once I was able to be honest with myself, using my past patterns as an example, the corrections were much easier to identify and implement.

My friend, however, found an entirely different set of struggles. He tried a multitude of ways to keep a Workout Journal on his own and nothing seemed to stick. Some methods had more longevity than others, but nothing foundational enough to sustain an entire program or even enough time to form any solid habits. He told me that it took a large toll on his emotional energy when it came to exercising, which was understandable considering the frustrations. As we learned earlier, you won't be fully and personally prepared for the journey unless every aspect of the program is taken into account. Maintaining the Workout Journal is just as imperative to your success as the workouts themselves! This was obvious when it came to my friend and his struggles.

When he finally took the time to sit down and hold himself

fully accountable, he was able to take that important breath and analyze the situation. His frustration was real, but when it became his focus there was no forward motion—no progress. Taking the time, he also reviewed old methods; even going back to his college coursework. What he discovered was that his best work and results came when he had more guidance throughout the process. That presented a large issue, as he was doing the workout individually due to scheduling and distance, so guidance was difficult to have consistently present. He considered using videos and webcam meetings to keep an outside form of guidance going, but he mentioned that he felt less motivated than ever.

This went on for several weeks and, through a few conversations, I was beginning to feel my friend's frustration. He had a tendency to take a classic approach to most things and it had usually worked out—no pun intended—but in this situation, I suggested taking a different angle to it. First, as with the entire program, it was vital that he was completely honest with himself. He always had willpower, and it was displayed in other aspects of his life. However, when it came to keeping a journal, there was difficulty. Then it was important to make sure to approach the solution from a place without judgement. He was feeling like he failed and that sense of failure was overwhelming. When there is so much negativity, it becomes increasingly difficult to overcome it when you are addressing it with the same approach. By taking a different perspective and applying new methods to the issue, you are expanding the possibility of a solution!

After a few days, my friend called me saying that he had indeed found a way that seemed to work. Intrigued, I asked what methods he ended up going with. He had gone to a local bookstore and found several journal-like guides to working out that gave him the parameters to measure ahead of time. He had never considered anything with a fill-in-the-blank theme for several reasons—he admitted it just seemed juvenile, he didn't put much stock in that style to help him, and that pride had held him back from expanding his thought process to include all methods. Within a day of having this guide, he felt energized and motivated to start the routines again! Not only did this book aid him during the program, but he was able to think outside his usual parameters. He has said that now, since that experience, he approaches his life with a different attitude—one of open thought and no judgement.

That has made all the difference!

With your Workout Journal in hand, you are one step closer to being completely prepared for this incredible journey! Celebrate another milestone in this process!

Chapter Summary

- Why are the first 30 days important?
- Forms correct habits
- A chance to identify problem areas early on
- This is a contract between you and yourself
- Why are the first 30 days important **to you**?
- Do not try and force yourself into the wrong workout
- The workout must fit you!
- Have you reviewed Chapter 6 for details on the upcoming workouts?
- List your past workout attempts
- Why didn't you follow through on those?
- What patterns do you see in relation to them ending?
- Are you being truly honest with yourself?

- Have you kept a Workout Journal before?
- Did it help with the process?
- Why or why not?
- Why is a Workout Journal important?
- What kind of Workout Journal is going to be most effective **for you**?

CHAPTER FIVE: DIET AND AVOIDING PITFALLS

Shortcuts are everywhere in life and they are becoming increasingly easy to find. The unfortunate reality is that the result has become exponentially more important than the journey. We want the finish line and when opportunities arise that promise us that sooner than others—or even just sooner than our previous time—it is incredibly tempting to jump at that chance.

We previously discussed both honesty and accountability with yourself and, as with your workouts themselves, we built upon previous knowledge to enhance the current task. Without the tools you've either discovered or honed, this moment will provide much more difficulty than necessary. Some of these "easy ways to win" are built on the assumption that you are not dedicated to the *journey* and would rather get to the end. This may have been the case in the past, but I know you are committed to your workout path and not just the desire to skip ahead! You have bettered yourself and it is going to pay off!

I have always been a firm believer in education for every

single situation. The more you know, the more ready you are when that part of life occurs. With this in mind, it is also important that you educate yourself on the kinds of shortcuts that could be temptations along the way.

Rather than tiptoe around an issue, I've always believed that meeting it directly is a much more effective choice. At no point in this journey should chemical alterations be brought into the mix! While for many this seems fairly obvious, there are times when a quick fix is enticing. The commercializing and ease of availability creates many problems when dealing with steroids and hormone treatments.

Despite the well-known downsides and potentially deadly side-effects of using these methods, the injuries, deaths, and various handicaps still happen because that end result takes up the entire view. The bottom line is straight-forward and should be adhered to: never use either!

During this process, as we've said before, you may decide to include a diet as well. While we do not provide one, finding a diet to fit the changes you are looking for is an excellent addition to your journey. That, and two other foundational variables will help you not only get the most out of this program, but form habits that will last!

Rest

The importance of rest cannot be overstated! In our fast-paced lifestyle, there is barely a moment to take three deep breaths, let alone get as much sleep as we need. You know the facts and you've known them for most of your life: 7-8 hours of sleep! The first thoughts you just had were most likely a list of reasons why that amount of sleep is rarely possible, if ever! That is a viable and real reason—life does not stop when you begin a program or make a change. Just like we made sure the importance of proper scheduling was stated, it is just as vital that you see proper sleep as an absolute as well.

By following the program, you will be taking time and effort to schedule your workouts to not only fit into your life, but improve it as well. This same method *must* be applied to your sleep schedule. You most likely have not made major alterations to your schedule in order to accommodate sleep; or if you have, they have been minimal. This time around, the changes will be real and lasting! Take some time now to go over the potential schedule you've been creating for the coming months and jot down how much sleep you think you will get each night. Remember, be honest! It does no good to make it look impressive on paper when you know the reality is not. Once you have seen the sleep you assume you will get laid out, begin finding adjustments you can make to add more sleep each night. There will not be a sudden opening that magically gives the time to keep your schedule as it is; there *will be* changes made!

Before moving on to the next foundational aspect, continue focusing on your sleep schedule. It is going to take some tinkering, so it is perfectly fine to bookmark this spot and finish before continuing.

Eating Habits

Just like every person will have a different approach to working out, the same applies to your eating habits during the program. Adapting to a new diet can require just as much effort as the workout regiment, but will also yield wonderful results. It is up to you how much you plan to alter your current diet and it largely depends on, again, your ability to be honest and direct with yourself. Take into consideration

CHAPTER FIVE: DIET AND AVOIDING PITFALLS

your current diet and general food habits when making this decision.

There are different approaches to creating a diet depending on the results you are looking for. Some people are looking to bulk up while they go through the program, while others prefer a more balanced approach across a larger range of varieties. The world of food and exercise are directly linked, and we'll cover the basics regarding the do's and don't's of a calisthenics diet. To help you create your own custom plan based around what works best for your schedule and budget, we'll cover two possible, specific diets—one for bulk and one based around calisthenics in general. You should feel free to consider this a buffet of knowledge. Pick through, find the things that will fit your journey, and commit to those changes!

One of the best things about calisthenics and its relationship to food is that it isn't complicated to follow! While there are detailed diets that relate very well to workouts—and we'll go over some of them—when you break it down, there are a few simple rules to follow; but the first and most important is that common sense will solve most questions you have. You already know most of what you need to know! It seems too easy, doesn't it?

One of the most common pitfalls people encounter when they begin creating a diet plan is that they have to relearn everything. This just isn't true! While there are some complexities that we will also cover, what you have learned about basic health and what foods are "good and bad" for you translate directly to this process! You have the control and are more than capable of creating a working diet for this journey!

Here are a few tips to get the ideas flowing! Take some time to review these before you start creating the actual plan.

- Take the time to get a better idea about where your current diet is. Over the course of a week—or whatever time frame will give you an idea of your patterns—keep track of your diet. Be as detailed as you would like. Remember, all of this information is for *your benefit*!
- Make notes where you see areas of improvement. After you have collected that data, review it to give yourself a wider view of your possible problem areas.
- Again, because it cannot be overstated, the more honest you are with yourself, the better chance you have to make real progress!
- "*In everything, moderation.*" By keeping this mantra in mind, you will already have an excellent guide to beginning the alterations to your diet. This simple rule applies to every part of life, but is especially true in regards to what you eat and drink. When you identify your problem areas in regards to food, moderate where you see excess. The most common excess is sugar, for example, in the daily lives of the average adult. By taking the correct steps early in the process, you will magnify your results and solidify those good habits!
- I really do not like when a program or diet refuses to take budget into account. It is a reality of life and should be taken seriously. While an ideal diet would consist almost entirely of organic foods, that is not always a possibility. Instead, find a few foods you enjoy that you can replace with an organic substitute—a few small changes will go a long way!

- A great place to start is with your fruit and vegetables. Find a local farmers' market or produce shop where you can discuss organic options with the growers themselves!
- When it comes to nutrition for a workout, nothing is more useful than protein! No matter what changes you make in your diet, it is imperative that the addition or increase of protein be top of the list. You can't replace or substitute for protein, especially when undertaking a program such as this. Depending on your personal preferences, you can supplement this with meat or another choice of yours.
- If you are including meat in your diet, to the best of your ability, focus on grass-fed animals and wild-caught fish products. You may experience the same budgetary restrictions when doing this; so again, focus on altering what you are able to. It is recommended to include between 0.6 grams to 1 gram of protein for every pound of body weight. As long as you are getting the necessary protein you are making the correct decisions!
- If you prefer not to include meat or fish, there are still plenty of sources to get that all-important protein from—tofu, edamame, chickpeas, lentils, hempseed, quinoa, or soy milk, just to name a few. By adding or increasing your intake of these products you will be taking the right steps towards your goal of betterment.

A vital part of the diet that isn't always addressed in these sections is the importance of hydration. This may seem redundant and unnecessary since everyone knows to drink water, right? That is partly true. Every person may *know* to drink water and properly hydrate, and yet we all know that few people actually follow through. It could be a matter of personal preference or just something you never really thought about. There are many times that common sense subjects such as this are incredibly interesting, considering the assumptions behind it. If everyone knows how to stay hydrated then everyone must be doing it, right? Wrong again, unfortunately.

Hydration is absolutely something you should include as part of your diet. Don't assume that you will just fall in line along the way and become a master of hydration; this simply isn't realistic. However, by putting that effort in and changing it from an assumed subject to a discussed subject, you give yourself all the power and possibility!

Do some research into the subject. What kind of hydration is recommended? Is water the only suitable choice? Are the water-energy additives harmful? These are exactly the kinds of questions you should be asking. Don't remove your personal preferences from the equation, as it is important to enjoy as much as you can. There are many more options than ever before to allow hydration to take a form you are more familiar with.

There are actually other ways than simply water to ensure you are properly hydrated. Did you know that?

Adding oatmeal to your diet will actually provide a great source of electrolytes and help aid your natural hydration!

If you are going for a diet that includes pasta, possibly consider replacing your usual pasta with a zucchini noodle. The zucchini noodle can be over 90% water and an incredibly fulfilling addition to any diet.

Choosing a low-sugar fruit smoothie option for a small snack can add that midday burst of energy you needed. Fruit smoothies, when the sugar isn't the main ingredient, are an excellent source of water and allow you that fun side as well.

Do you have frozen fruit? While fruit in general provides excellent hydration, freezing them can, once thawed, create even more chances to increase your health and continue bettering your life!

Be flexible in all your thinking, even on how to get the right amount of water. You'll probably be surprised by the options available to you with just a little research!

These two foundational parts—proper sleep and diet—of the workout journey will be invaluable tools as you move forward! They are more than just variables in the process. By maintaining the habits you are learning here, you will have gained invaluable knowledge and trust between yourself and the depth of this program. There is a third and final foundational principle before you get to The Ultimate Calisthenics Workout in the next chapter.

The Workout

We have covered a wide array of tools, techniques, and troubleshooting that will be vital during the program—the Workout Journal, self-awareness, honesty, and accountability of self, to name a few. While these are all important, we broke it down into three key factors that, when customized to your schedule and adhered to, will be foundational paths to success! We reviewed both proper sleep habits and diet, but the third is one that you have actually been learning along the way this entire time: the workout itself!

There is no middle ground for this subject. As we discussed earlier, many workout routines have a singular approach; and even if they touch on a variety of areas, it is from a surface perspective and rarely offers in-depth solutions or tools to better oneself. When considering the possible variables that would help build this program, it became apparent very early on that by only adhering to one or two of the three keys, you create a problem area rather than solving one. The design includes all three in order to ensure the changes are lasting and the altered life you have formed will not falter.

This cannot be overemphasized! While other sections are more of a buffet-style that allows you to pick and choose, this requires a stricter adherence. You *must* give the same focus to sleep, diet, and workout. An imbalance will prove incredibly disruptive down the line, even if you don't see it right now. By taking the time early into the program and solidifying the perspectives you will be coming from, you are making that all-important investment in yourself. That's one that will certainly pay huge dividends! By beginning from a place of detail and focusing on changing your habits, you have readied yourself for the challenges ahead. To truly bring about change—*real change*—in your life, it takes all three factors! If you allow that honesty to yourself, then it has become apparent why past attempts had faltered and burned out. We've been able to look at these reasons not as failures, but as chances to get better and learn where our life alterations needed to happen.

Most programs have a tendency to put a disproportionate focus on the workouts and leave the other two factors on the backburner. By doing this, the habits you develop are lopsided. You'll find yourself trying to address proper rest when you're halfway through the second month, or you'll become stressed by struggling to alter your diet without putting the proper time and thought into it before reaching the halfway point. It's harder to change the rules when you're

CHAPTER FIVE: DIET AND AVOIDING PITFALLS

in the middle of the game. This just means to build those habits the correct, balanced way. Empower yourself for those difficult moments down the road—ones you probably haven't even considered! The first two keys give you the extra energy and time to give your effort where it should be: your workouts.

Every day of the program—and maintaining it afterwards—is built on reminding yourself of those three factors. This can be made easier by putting it into the form of three questions that are part of beginning your day:

1. Do I feel rested?
2. Will my diet for today help me succeed?
3. Have I familiarized myself with my workouts for today?

Everyone knows that starting your day correctly will help create a more balanced and aware daily life. These three baseline questions to yourself will give you a readiness right out of the gate! Also, take this chance to customize your *Readiness Questions* so you feel motivated and excited about the new day before you! I speak out loud when I ask myself these questions in the morning, others have a motivational reminder beside the bed or in the bathroom, and some find entirely new ways of going about it. The bottom line is that up to now you have found ways to make this journey truly yours—a custom path that does not disrupt your life, but rather flows through and enriches it. Do the same here.

That was a large and important section to cover there. Do you feel like you absorbed it all? There is a massive amount of information in this program, and each piece is designed to bring the best out of you. If there is ever a time you seem confused or less than sure of why or how to implement one of these betterment chances, take the time to keep investing in yourself. Reread sections if needed, or sometimes hearing a section out loud alters the way you take in that information. The bottom line is to not worry about changing things up. Flexibility where it can be utilized will make the entire experience all the more personal.

When dealing with the possible problems and pitfalls that come with a workout commitment, there is still one important thing to cover: where you went wrong before.

Take that all-important breath and return to that judgement-free place. There are no attacks here, simply direct confrontations. You've taken time in previous sections to think upon and even list your past workout attempts in order to identify problem patterns. We were able to skim and collect data that has proved invaluable! In the best method for your productivity, single out the specific problem areas you encountered in the past and this time don't avoid detail. These pinpointed problem areas will lead to what we call your *Problem Journey*. Just as this process is a journey of betterment, the past times it just didn't work ended up creating a journey as well—one of negativity and a lack of confidence. You have probably been harder on yourself than you needed to be; and as that compiled, it weighed you down more and more until the mere idea of starting a routine up again carries no motivation. It simply brings back memories of not following through.

Here is a vital place in your journey where you can alter the perspective you naturally take. As you go over the list you made and map out the ways you hit the road blocks and difficulties, be sure to notice why you ended up stopping altogether. Now compare that to the ongoing notes you've kept in regards to the positive steps you recognized during this time around. You'll find that, more often than not, you are solving old issues you have had without even realizing it.

Many people starting out include others in their routines. Really take a look and see if this occurred and did it bring about distraction or worse? That is not a judgement on yourself or the partner(s) you chose for that workout. Some people work better when the accountability is with them and another person, but this system is designed to nurture honesty with yourself.

Perhaps you let early schedule disruptions fill you with a feeling of being overwhelmed. You may see now that you've managed to take the disruptions in stride and alter your schedule to smoothly keep your responsibilities and still work out.

On the other hand, maybe your issue was pushing way too hard in the beginning and you strained yourself, gave yourself extended time to recover, and just never started up again. Well, this time you were able to be honest with yourself and crafted a schedule with your physical limits in mind.

Another possible reason is what I call "the allure of equipment"! The amount of unused exercise equipment sitting in rooms across the country is staggering. If every person who bought a treadmill or stationary bike followed through on those commitments, there would be no health issues regarding working out! Unfortunately, this is far from the case. The promise that tends to come with these machines is usually overstated and comes with a slew of fine print; and nothing good ever comes filled with fine print! As you learned prior, you will be relying on you and your bodyweight to be all the equipment you need. A little imagination, and suddenly you don't need some elaborate mechanism to inspire you—you have become your own muse!

No matter what the problem is, you will keep finding solutions to issues and pitfalls you had encountered previously as you continue through the program! These are just the beginnings to the positive changes you are well on your way to bringing about!

Chapter Summary

- Are you focused on the results or the journey?
- Avoid bringing chemicals into the mix?
- Hormones and steroids are harmful and will not create a positive result
- How much sleep do you get per night?
- Do you feel rested or energized?
- Does your schedule reflect a balanced focus on sleep as well?
- Are you still being honest with yourself?
- What changes need to be made to your diet?
- Will you be using a specific diet in collaboration with the program?
- Is your diet currently where you want it to be?
- Have you taken your budget into account when planning your dietary changes?
- Are you starting your day with the three *Readiness Questions*?
- Do I feel rested?
- Will my diet for today help me succeed?
- Have I familiarized myself with my workouts for today?
- Are you holding yourself accountable daily?

CHAPTER SIX: THE ULTIMATE CALISTHENICS WORKOUT

As you've no doubt noticed, there is a great deal of focus on celebrating moments and goals in this program. This is a big one! You have gone through some very honest times to get to this point, and for that you should be incredibly proud of yourself! There were moments in which you were asked to be very direct and self-aware, all of which you took on and not only utilized, but have now truly prepared you for the rest of this journey!

The key to your progress up to now has been preparedness in all aspects. By taking the time to increase your self-awareness, you have built an armory of knowledge all before even lifting a finger! You should be familiar with the upcoming workouts in a general sense; and thanks to your adherence to scheduling, you enter this phase without the worry of the unknown.

These are the last few moments before the actual physical portion will begin; so take the time, as we do, to review your preparedness to this point.

In Chapters 1 and 2 we gave you a brief overview of what you could expect from the workout routines and the schedule you would be keeping. Now the program will be fleshed out and you will be able to start this incredible journey!

Before you move ahead and begin the actual routines, take some time and review the tips and foundational keys for your workouts. When you start that first exercise it should be from a place of peace and preparedness. Any feelings of being unsure should not be ignored. By now, you have become pretty comfortable with self-honesty, so do a self-review now to see if anything seems off or is a lingering bother. Maybe there was one day in your schedule that just seemed overly stressful to maintain, or you need to do a check on groceries to ensure you can follow your chosen diet without distress. As discussed, these are all real and important aspects of this journey and should be recognized and fixed.

There is no need to rush through these last self checks. It is much more beneficial to address any possible pitfalls now rather than attempting to adjust when it could have been prevented.

You know yourself, so don't over-analyze the situation. If you feel comfortable and ready, which you certainly are, then you are welcomed to The Ultimate Calisthenics Workout!

Month 1 - Full Body 101

Here are the exercises, form, and methods you will be doing during the first four-week cycle:

Running In Place [Works the quads, calf muscles, hamstrings, glutes, and hip flexors]: Use a steady pace. Knees maintain a smooth motion. This is an excellent warmup. Control your breathing, avoiding sharp breaths or halting breathing. Try to avoid jarring motions when your feet strike the floor. Keep the movements smooth to avoid undue pressure on your joints.

Squats [Works the abdominals, calves, glutes, quads, and hamstrings]: Use your legs, not your back. Feet slider wider than your hips. As you go into the squat position, work your hips backwards into the sit. Keep both of your entire feet on the ground. To stand, push from your heels and straighten your legs. Avoid jerking motions; instead aim for smooth movement.

Push Ups [Works the pectorals, shoulders, triceps, and abdominals]: For an effective push up, your form is much more important than speed or quantity. View your body as a plank—unbending from heel to head. Hands shoulder-width apart. As you begin the push up, keep your elbows at a 45 degree angle from your body. Adjust for comfort. Lower to about an inch from the ground and, in a smooth motion, extend your elbows to push back to the starting position.

Knee Raises [Works the hamstrings, quads, glutes, and calves]: Lay flat on your back with your arms to your side and your legs straightened and together. In one smooth motion, pull both knees from the floor towards your chest. Exhale as you let your legs straighten back to lying straight.

Chair Dips [Works the triceps]: The preferred method is to use a **solid** chair for this exercise, but a bottom stair or a raised, level area will work just as well. So long as you ensure your form and motions are correct, you will get the most out of this exercise!

Sit normally on a **sturdy** chair (or desired option). Grip the front of the chair on either outer side of your legs. Shift yourself up onto your hands and shift your body forward. Your feet can scoot forward to help you, knees bent. When you are hovering, lower yourself by bending your elbows, breathing in. Exhale as you push yourself back up. If you feel uneasy, go back to sitting position and try a better angle.

Follow this guide for sets and repetitions:

- **Running In Place:** 3 minutes
- **Squats:** 2 sets of 10
- **Push Ups:** 3 sets of 5
- **Knee Raises:** 3 sets of 5
- **Chair Dips:** 3 sets of 5

If you find that you need more of a challenge—give yourself at least one session before deciding—you can add a set to each routine. Track how you feel from this increase and ensure that you are not pushing yourself too hard. As this is the first month, avoid putting unneeded stress on yourself. You are laying a foundation here and by expecting a journey rather than a sprint, you can better prepare yourself for the basics you have learned here.

This is the first month and your focus needs to be on correct form and following the guide laid out in Chapter 4. As a reminder, here is your schedule guideline for **Full Body 101**:

- Day 1: Full Body 101
- Day 2: Rest
- Day 3: Full Body 101
- Day 4: Rest
- Day 5: Full Body 101
- Day 6: Rest
- Day 7: Full Body 101

CHAPTER SIX: THE ULTIMATE CALISTHENICS WORKOUT

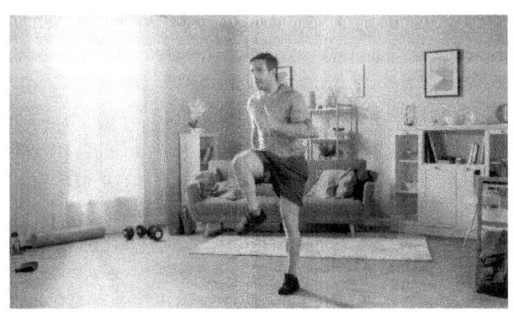

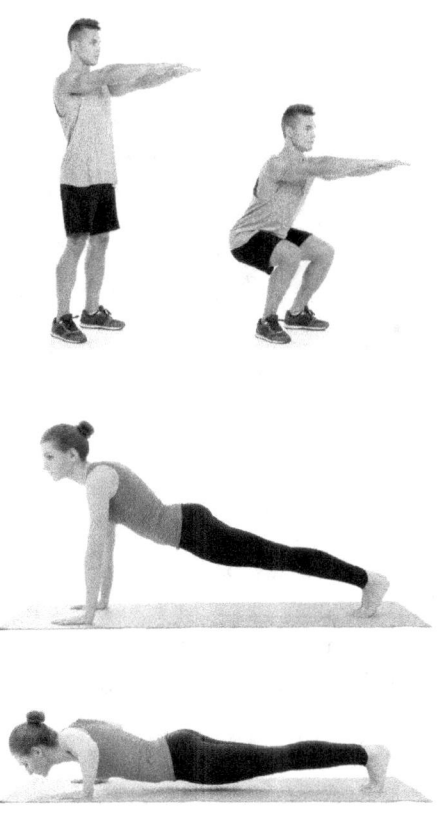

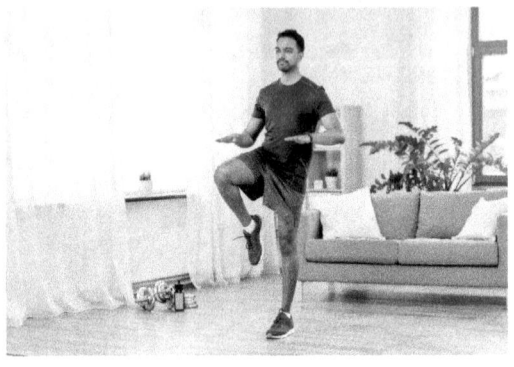

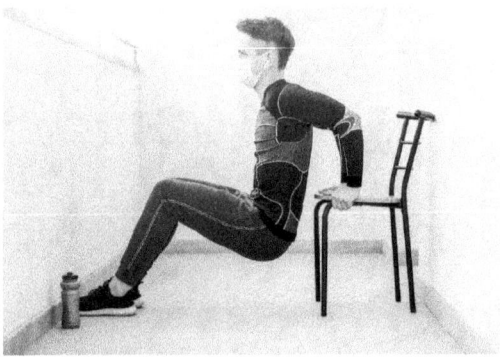

Month 2 - Full Body 102

This month will give focus to a wider range of muscle groups. Month 1 began giving you the tools to create a solid foundation; and in this month, you will be building upwards and adding in more impact on core muscle groups.

Here are the exercises you will be doing during this four-week cycle:

Running In Place [Works the quads, calf muscles, hamstrings, glutes, and hip flexors]: See **Full Body 101**

Lunges [Works the hamstrings, glutes, and quads]: Stand feet shoulder-width apart. Taking a large step forward, ensure your heel lands first. Lower your body until your lower knee barely touches the ground. Push back from the heel to go back into standing form.

Decline Push Ups [Works the upper chest, pectorals]: For this exercise, the best method is to use a low stool or bottom step. Use the same proper push up form that you learned in **Full Body 101** but with your feet up on the raised surface. Lower yourself in push up form, straightening your elbows to rise back up.

Standing Leg Raises [Works the abdominals and hip flexors]: Standing feet shoulder-width apart, lift one leg straight forward and up in a slow, direct motion. Hold for a 2-count, exhale while lowering the leg to the ground. Avoid bending your knee at any time during the exercise.

Reverse Row [Works the trapezius, biceps, and back]: This is an exercise that will be modified later on, so ensure your basic form is correct.

For this exercise the best way is to be underneath a **sturdy** table. The height should be 6-10 inches from the tips of your fingers, lying underneath, arm pointed upwards. Once you have a **strong** table or similar surface, position yourself underneath shoulders aligned with the table edge above you.

Raise your arms and bend at the waist upwards until you can firmly grip the edge of the table. Using a surface with a low slip-possibility is best. Your body is your counterweight as you bend your elbows, pulling yourself up towards the table. Breathe in while going up, exhaling while straightening your elbows back to original form. Be cautious not to drop yourself to avoid injury!

Follow this guide for sets and repetitions:

- **Running In Place:** 5 minutes
- **Lunges:** 2 sets of 10
- **Decline Push Ups:** 3 sets of 5
- **Standing Leg Raises:** 3 sets of 10
- **Reverse Row:** 3 sets of 5

If you find that you need more of a challenge—give yourself at least one session before deciding—you can add a set to each routine. Track how you feel from this increase and ensure you are not pushing yourself too hard.

For the second month you will be following this schedule guideline:

- Day 1: Full Body 102
- Day 2: Rest
- Day 3: Full Body 102
- Day 4: Rest
- Day 5: Full Body 102
- Day 6: Rest
- Day 7: Full Body 102

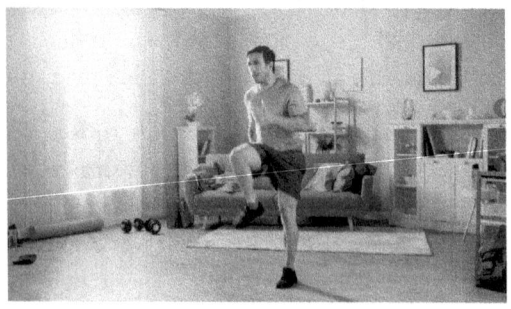

CHAPTER SIX: THE ULTIMATE CALISTHENICS WORKOUT

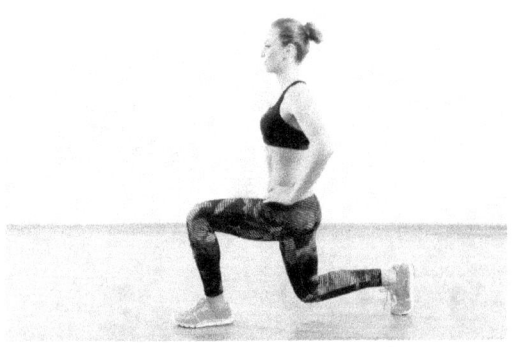

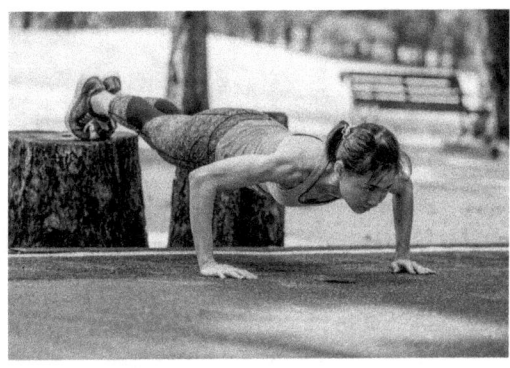

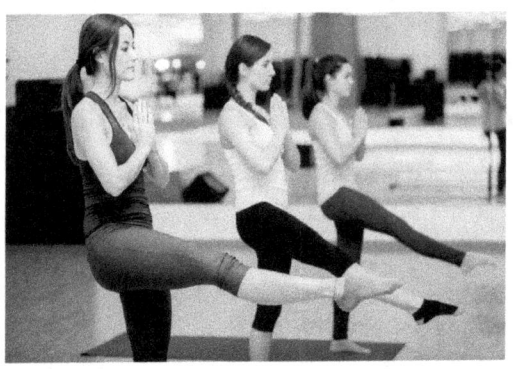

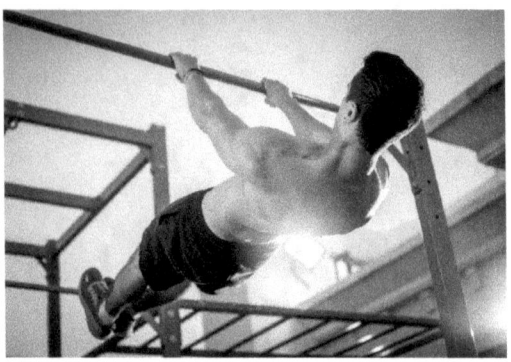

Month 3 - Intermediate 101

As you progress further into the program, take note of any tightness or strain into pain that you have felt. You may need to incorporate a minute or two of stretching to help with those more complex routines. If you do feel that pull of tightness, do not try and push past it. You may hyperextend or tear a muscle. Avoid injury at all costs. Stretching is an easy way to avoid these pitfalls.

Here are the exercises you will be doing for the next four-week cycle:

Running In Place [Works the quads, calf muscles, hamstrings, glutes, and hip flexors]: See **Full Body 101**

Duck Walk [Works the thighs, lower legs, and glutes]: Stand feet shoulder-width apart. Lower yourself into a squat and then lower your buttocks so your knees are bent in front of you. Keep your feet flat on the ground. If you are having balance problems, use your arms to the sides and front to help. Staying as low as you can—avoid overextending your knees and lower back—step forward, and in a waddle-like motion, step with the other foot.

Calf Raises [Works the hamstrings and calves]: On a step or raised area, stand with your heels off the edge of the step (or desired option) and the rest of your feet flat on the step. Inhaling, raise your heels up until you are on, or as close to as is comfortable, your tiptoes. Exhale as you lower your heels down until your feet are back to the flat, original form.

Be aware of your surroundings when doing this exercise as you will be facing up the stairs, if that is your desired option. Avoid injury!

Higher Decline Push Ups [Works the upper chest, pectorals]: You will be using the same push up form that you have learned to this point. Use a raised area that is higher than the one used in **Decline Push Ups**. Perform the correct form for a push up to complete the sets.

Back-Bridge Push Ups [Works the hip abductors, glutes, hamstrings, and erector spinae (length of the spinal cord)]: Unlike most of the other exercises you have done to this point, there is extra caution to be taken when approaching this particular one. Your flexibility has most likely improved by this point in the program, but this specific angle and form may be stretching in a way you are not used to. Because of this, take time to build up to full form. Do not be discouraged if your initial, and even first few, attempts are not as refined or with the same ease that you have with the other exercises.

To start, lie flat on the ground and stretch your arms and legs away from your body. You should feel the stretch in your joints. Now with your torso still flat, shift your legs until your knees are pointing up and your feet are flat on the ground. Do the same with your arms—elbows pointing up, palms as flat as possible.

Again, this seems extremely complex; but after a few times, the form will be more understood and your muscles will loosen.

From that position, push from your palms and feet, arching your back in the air. Do not push yourself past a point of pain. It should burn, not hurt. Once you reach your apex, exhale as you lower your torso back to the ground in a smooth motion.

Follow this guide for sets and repetitions:

- **Running In Place:** 5 minutes
- **Duck Walk:** Forward 10 steps, backwards 10 steps. 2 reps
- **Calf Raises:** 3 sets of 5
- **High Decline Push Ups:** 3 sets of 5
- **Back-Bridge Push Ups:** 2 sets of 5

If you find that you need more of a challenge—give yourself at least one session before deciding—you can add a set to each routine. Track how you feel from this increase and ensure you are not pushing yourself too hard.

Here is your schedule guideline for the third month:

- Low-Impact Schedule:
- Day 1: Intermediate 101
- Day 2: Rest
- Day 3: Intermediate 101
- Day 4: Rest
- Day 5: Intermediate 101
- Day 6: Rest

- Day 7: Intermediate 101
- High-Impact Schedule:
- Day 1: Intermediate 101
- Day 2: Rest
- Day 3: Intermediate 101
- Day 4: Light Running
- Day 5: Intermediate 101
- Day 6: Light Running
- Day 7: Rest

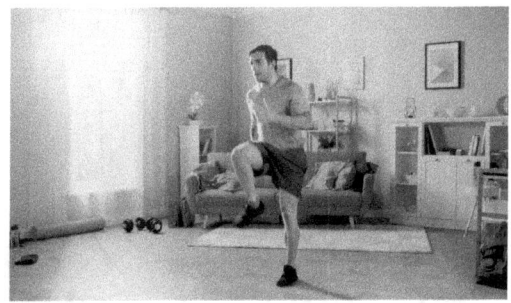

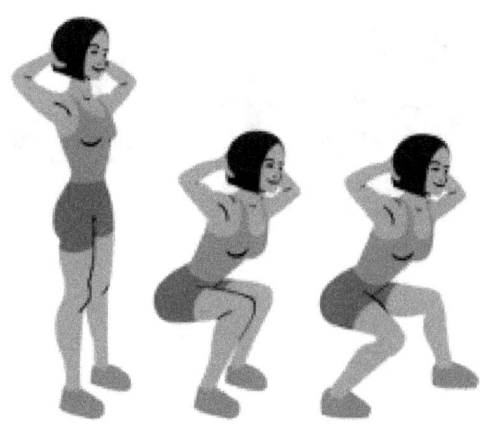

DUCK WALKS

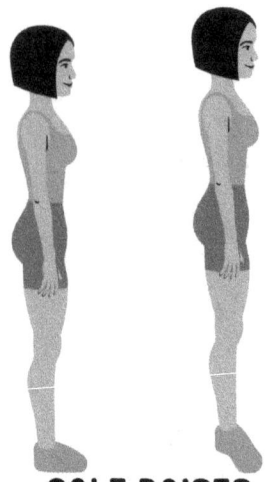

CALF RAISES

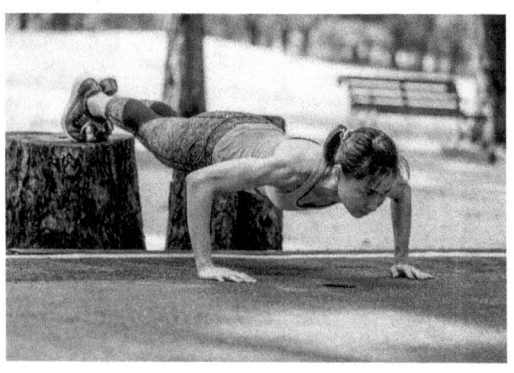

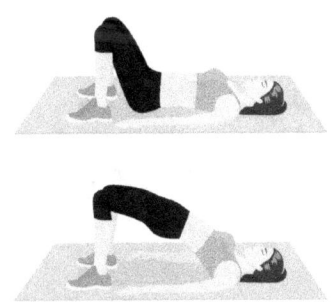

Month 4 - Muscle Impact 101

For the next four-week cycle, here are the exercises you will be doing:

Running In Place [Works the quads, calf muscles, hamstrings, glutes, and hip flexors]: See **Full Body 101**

Horizontal Jump [Works the hip flexors, glutes, quads, abs, calves, and hamstrings]: Stand feet shoulder-width apart. With your arms up, stretched, rise onto the balls of your feet. As you bring your arms behind you, rock slightly forward, then raise your arms as you stand. Repeat several times to prepare. Arms, behind, rock slightly, then drive your feet down and push to jump, your arms moving forward. Make sure to land flat-footed in a smooth motion.

Mountain Climbers [Works the glutes, shoulders, triceps, full legs, and abdominals]: Use the plank-like form to begin —back straight. Bend one knee inwards, towards your front. In a smooth motion, bring the leg back and return to original form. Bend the other knee inwards, and in the same smooth motion, return to form.

**Reverse Row Dips [Works the trapezius, biceps, and

back]: Using the same method in form you used for **Reverse Row**. This time reverse the form so your head is the only thing under the table, your legs and torso out from underneath. Reach up and reverse grip the table edge. Bend at the waist until you have a firm hold. Like a pull-up, keep your body straight as you pull yourself up (inhaling) and lower yourself (exhaling) in a smooth motion.

Take caution to not drop yourself to avoid injury!

Reverse Row Leg Raises [Works the trapezius, biceps, hamstrings, glutes, and back]: Use the same reverse form from **Reverse Row Dips**. Rather than lifting yourself, grip the edge of the table, focusing on your abs and core, raise one straight leg and hold for a 5-count. Release and lower your leg in a smooth motion.

Follow this guide for sets and repetitions:

- **Running In Place:** 5 minutes
- **Horizontal Jump:** 3 sets of 5
- **Mountain Climbers:** 3 minutes
- **Reverse Row Dips:** 3 sets of 5
- **Reverse Row Leg Raises:** 3 sets of 5, alternating legs, 3 sets per leg

If you find that you need more of a challenge—give yourself at least one session before deciding—you can add a set to each routine. Track how you feel from this increase and ensure you are not pushing yourself too hard.

Here is your schedule guideline for the fourth month:

- Day 1: Muscle Impact 101
- Day 2: Rest
- Day 3: Muscle Impact 101

- Day 4: Rest
- Day 5: Muscle Impact 101
- Day 6: Rest
- Day 7: Light Running

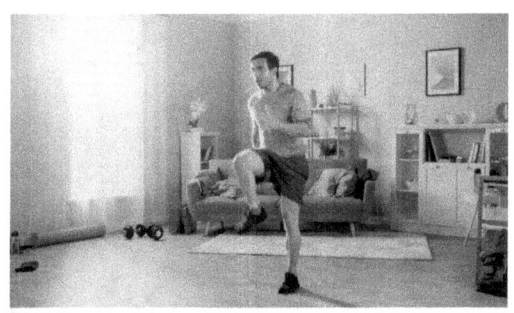

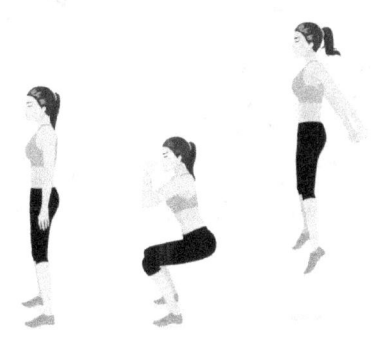

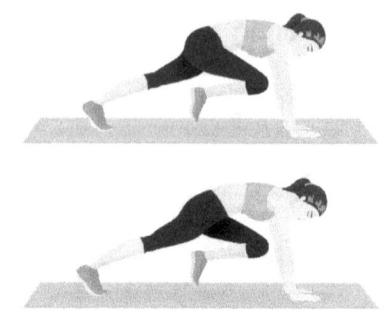

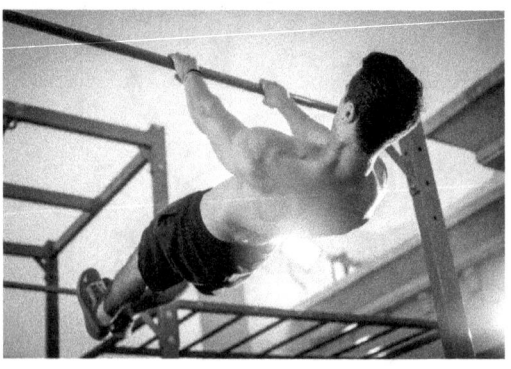

Month 5 - Muscle Impact 102

For this month, you will begin interspersing previous routines into your schedule. While you *will* be learning new exercises, we will be referring to older routines to help continue your amazing forward progress! Make sure to take the time and review the exercises and form you used for the routines we are doing again. You have kept excellent notes and this is exactly why!

For the fifth month four-week cycle here are the exercises, you will be doing:

Running In Place [Works the quads, calf muscles, hamstrings, glutes, and hip flexors]: See **Full Body 101**

Jumping Jacks [Works the calves, glutes, and thighs]: You are probably familiar with this exercise. Rather than just trying to get through it, focus on the form and the smooth motions. As a child, there was probably flailing involved, so let's get it right this time around!

Vertical Jump [Works the hamstrings, quads, calves, and glutes]: Start from a standing position, legs shoulder-width apart. Stretch slightly by lowering yourself slowly into a squat, then back to standing. After repeating this a few times, you are ready for the jump. Lower yourself from the standing position a level slightly lower than a typical squat. You should feel the stretch in your thighs. Pressing from the balls of your feet, spring upwards, pointing your toes as you jump. Keep a smooth motion, avoid locking your knees, and avoid any jerking motion. You may also want to draw shorter breaths—avoid this by breathing fully during stretches.

Reverse Row Leg Raises [Works the trapezius, biceps, hamstrings, glutes, and back]: See **Muscle Impact 101**

Chin Hold Reverse Row [Works the trapezius, biceps, and back]: For this exercise, you will be using the same, under-the-table form from **Reverse Rows**. This is an advanced version of that routine, so ensure that your grip is non-slip and you are using extreme caution to avoid injury!

With your shoulders and head out from under the table, your torso and legs underneath, bend at the waist until you can firmly grip the edge of the table. Like in **Reverse Rows**, you will pull yourself upwards; but the goal with this exercise is to get your chin above the table edge. Do not push yourself past pain or if you feel unsure! Work your way until you find that level of comfort. Once you reach the apex, hold for 2-3 seconds, then exhale as you lower yourself to the ground.

Follow this guide for sets and repetitions:

- **Running In Place:** 5 minutes
- **Jumping Jacks:** 3 minutes
- **Vertical Jump:** 3 sets of 5
- **Reverse Row Leg Raises:** 3 sets of 5, alternating legs, 3 sets per leg
- **Chin Hold Reverse Row:** 3 sets of 5

If you find that you need more of a challenge—give yourself at least one session before deciding—you can add a set to each routine. Track how you feel from this increase and ensure you are not pushing yourself too hard.

Here is your schedule guideline for the fifth month:

- Day 1: Muscle Impact 102
- Day 2: Intermediate 101
- Day 3: Rest
- Day 4: Muscle Impact 102
- Day 5: Intermediate 101
- Day 6: Rest
- Day 7: Light Running

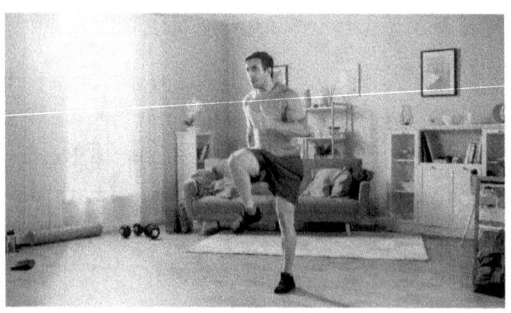

CHAPTER SIX: THE ULTIMATE CALISTHENICS WORKOUT

Jumping Jacks

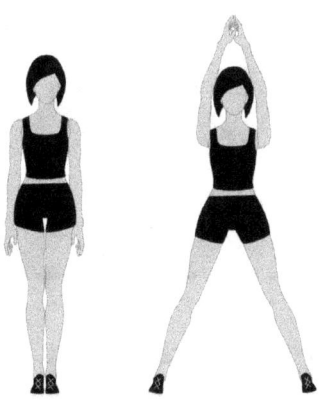

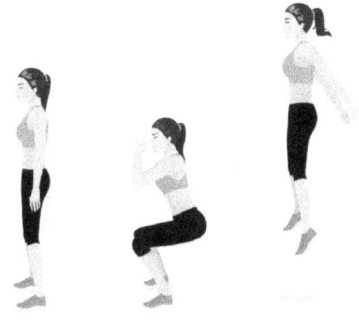

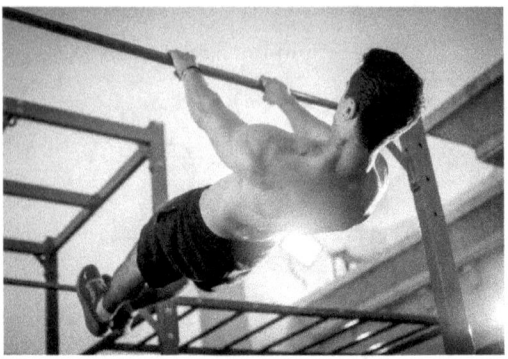

Month 6 - The Ultimate Calisthenics Workout

Here we are—the last month in the program! You should be both ecstatic and incredibly proud of yourself! Not only did you accomplish physical goals, but you have learned invaluable tools that are sure to stay with you long after you complete the final month!

Before you begin this last four-week cycle, take the time to do what we do best: review! By going back and seeing the progress you've made, you will get a broader, fuller understanding of just how much your journey has changed. You will be referring back to various routines that have made up your schedule to this point, as well as adding one day of high intensity!

The main addition to this final month is The Ultimate Calisthenics workout. This is a compilation of various muscle impact exercises that will give you that big push. You are more than ready and capable for this next step!

For the sixth month, here are the exercises you will be doing:

The Ultimate Calisthenics Workout

- 5 minutes Running In Place
- **[Works the quads, calf muscles, hamstrings, glutes, and hip flexors]**
- 5 Reverse Row Leg Raises
- **[Works the trapezius, biceps, hamstrings, glutes, and back]**
- 10 Reverse Rows
- **[Works the trapezius, biceps, and back]**
- 15 Push Ups
- **[Works the pectorals, shoulders, triceps, and abdominals]**
- 15 Decline Push Ups
- **[Works the upper chest, pectorals]**
- 10 Squats
- **[Works the abdominals, calves, glutes, quads, and hamstrings]**
- 3 minutes Running in Place

The first time you go through this workout, take some extra time to ensure you do not rush! The combination of these workouts bring about the best results, so the more detailed you are in form and movement the better! Be patient with yourself and focus on the individual sets rather than the entire routine.

As with **Muscle Impact 102**, you will be using previous routines blended into your schedule. It is a higher impact schedule than the previous five months, so if at any time you need to take a moment, do that! You need to feel comfortable with the motions, and you have given yourself all the tools to succeed. Because many of these exercises are ones you have done in past months, you can refer back to your Workout Journal at any time to ensure you get the most efficiency out of every movement.

Here is your schedule guideline for the sixth, and final, month:

- <u>Day 1</u>: Muscle Impact 101
- <u>Day 2</u>: Muscle Impact 102
- <u>Day 3</u>: Rest
- <u>Day 4</u>: Muscle Impact 102
- <u>Day 5</u>: Light Running
- <u>Day 6</u>: The Ultimate Calisthenics Workout
- <u>Day 7</u>: Rest

AT THIS MOMENT you should be basking in exhilaration! What you just accomplished is something that should be celebrated continuously and is a goal you've had in sight for six months! You took on a commitment and, for maybe the first time in your life, you have followed through on a workout routine. Say that out loud to yourself, even if it is just once:

"I have successfully completed a workout routine!"

The first time I got to say that felt incredible! There is something to be said about the power behind vocalizing a moment. As you finished your last rep and tidied up your area, it may not have hit you. Even when you turned out the light and walked away, it still might have barely registered. For me, it hit when I sat down to fill in my workout summary for the day and I saw the date and the schedule; and for the first time, there wasn't a next page. That is a big moment.

You may feel intimidated by that last statement, and it is a scary moment as well. There is no next page. It holds such a sense of finality that I am sure you feel the need to shift that perspective. Yes, something has finished and it *should* be recognized. However, it is not as much a closed door as you entering an entirely new hallway with a brand new set of doors. By completing this program and gaining the knowledge and ability that you have, life itself has actually been altered for you as well. Six months ago, your mindset and thought process were drastically different than the positive, confident, healthier you that exists now.

Before you completely move forward and begin the cool down portion of the program you, should take another moment. Thank your past self. I always prefer these moments to be vocal—it's between you and you after all—but your methods have worked for you to this point, so do not begin doubting them now. However you go about it, just thank that past version of yourself. It is easy to be hard on that person because you have the hindsight and experience to recognize the issues that need to be bettered, but you were not less of a person! In fact, you were an incredibly strong version of yourself because, despite being on that side of the spectrum, you took the step and began the process! There was no absolute assurance or magic ball to see what the future held; but you trusted and kept faith throughout! That, in a time in history where speed and results are the sole focus, you were patient and let the journey create growth. It is because of all this that your past self deserves your thanks and appreciation. From this point forward, because of that decision, you are better and shall continue to progress to heights that you can't even imagine yet.

"Thank you, past self."

Chapter Summary

- Have you taken the time and reviewed the tips and foundational keys for success?
- What day is going to begin your workout schedule?
- What muscle groups will be worked on in Month 1?
- Month 1 - Full Body 101
- Running In Place - 3 minutes
- Squats - 2 sets of 10
- Push Ups - 3 sets of 5
- Knee Raises - 3 sets of 5
- Chair Dips - 3 sets of 5
- Review your schedule for Full Body 101
- What muscle groups will be worked on in Month 2?
- Month 2 - Full Body 102
- Running In Place - 5 minutes
- Lunges - 2 sets of 10
- Decline Push Ups - 3 sets of 5
- Standing Leg Raises - 3 sets of 10
- Reverse Row - 3 sets of 5
- Review your schedule for Full Body 102
- What muscle groups will be worked on in Month 3?
- Month 3 - Intermediate 101
- Running In Place - 5 minutes
- Duck Walk - Forward 10 steps, backwards 10 steps, 2 reps
- Calf Raises - 3 sets of 5
- Higher Decline Push Ups - 3 sets of 5
- Back-Bridge Push Ups - 2 sets of 5
- Review your schedule for Intermediate 101
- Did you choose High or Low Impact?
- Review the first 3 months of progress
- What changes can you see so far?
- How has your sleep improved?

CHAPTER SIX: THE ULTIMATE CALISTHENICS WORKOUT

- What aspect of your personal life has improved the most?
- What muscle groups will be worked on in Month 4?
- Month 4 - Muscle Impact 101
- Running In Place - 5 minutes
- Horizontal Jump - 3 sets of 5
- Mountain Climbers - 3 minutes
- Reverse Row Dips - 3 sets of 5
- Reverse Row Leg Raises - 3 sets of 5, alternating legs, 3 sets per leg
- Review your schedule for Muscle Impact 101
- Have you previewed the changes from last month into Month 5?
- Are there any schedule changes you are uneasy about?
- What actions are you taking to rectify those issues?
- What muscle groups will be worked on in Month 5?
- Month 5 - Muscle Impact 102
- Running In Place - 5 minutes
- Jumping Jacks - 3 minutes
- Vertical Jump - 3 sets of 5
- Reverse Row Leg Raises - 3 sets of 5, alternating legs, 3 sets per leg
- Chin Hold Reverse Row - 3 sets of 5
- Preview the final month to recognize and address any uneasiness
- All muscle groups will be worked in Month 6
- Month 6 - The Ultimate Calisthenics Workout
- Running In Place - 5 minutes
- 5 Reverse Row Leg Raises
- 10 Reverse Rows
- 15 Push Ups
- 15 Decline Push Ups
- 10 Squats

- Running In Place - 3 minutes
- Are you rushing through The Ultimate Calisthenics Workout?
- Are you maintaining focus on your form despite the increase in intensity and impact?

CHAPTER SEVEN: WHEN PROBLEMS ARISE

As much as we would like a perfect world, the reality is that life becomes difficult sometimes. Unexpected events can disrupt any routine or commitment and it is not just an excuse, but a valid reason for that disruption. It may seem like a harsh word, but it describes what occurs quite perfectly—it is a hiccup, those roadblocks we have been discussing. An issue or scheduling problem can easily become a distraction, and from there it can take hold and begin throwing off your daily life and the new changes that come with it and become a disruption. It is vital to address these issues as they arise because, faster than you think, a disruption will lead to a complete derailment of the entire program.

Issue into distraction, distraction into disruption, disruption leads to derailment. The ability to repair these lies with you!

This journey that you have undertaken will be no different and, as such, is subject to possible distraction that creates the potential for disruption. Rather than press onward without truly taking that into consideration, let's take a moment and discuss the possible upcoming issues.

You have created a welcoming environment that is founded in honesty. There has been much asked of you and you have not only risen to the challenges, but excelled. Because of this, you have a distinct advantage when approaching problems in this program. When an issue comes about, rather than imploding or reacting with sudden impulse, you can breathe and know that this is not unexpected. These difficulties that derailed your past attempts are now dwarfed by perspective and trust. That is a valuable weapon against doubt! You wield personal experience and a plethora of knowledge at the ready and you enter each day and each session with readiness.

First and foremost, you must approach this section with the same lack of judgement that you have kept thus far. The subject of troubleshooting can bring up complications in that area, but know that you have a full handle on this! You've picked up tools that you can put to use whenever these road bumps occur. You have thanked your past self and from that you can continue to pull away from seeing that past in a negative light. The lack of judgement doesn't just apply to the present, but rather it extends backwards and forwards. Forgive yourself for the errors and derailments in the past, and trust that you will continue forward in that same vein of thought.

Scheduling

The most common instance where distraction can be planted and grow into the routine withering away is scheduling. By this point, you should be fairly protective of your schedule. We spent a considerable amount of time making sure the importance of proper scheduling is given to this commitment, and it was for a very good reason. Armed with a well-thought out and functional schedule, one that incorporates and promotes fluidity in the face of adversity, you are multiple steps ahead of every situation. Each time you move forward in the same spirit you strengthen that resolve!

Your life is a daily whirl of activity and events, so timing and properly blocking out days plays a huge role in ensuring you can succeed! You put considerable effort into creating a functional schedule for this workout program and it is worth standing up for!

When an issue does arise, the first thing you should do is be honest about the priority of the disruption to the schedule. It could be absolutely legitimate and is a responsibility that is yours alone, and for that you must put the same effort into altering your schedule. It is incredibly easy to shrug off a workout day as a knee-jerk response, but that becomes dangerously easier the more it occurs. See every moment as an individual event and give it the focus that deserves. You know your commitments that existed prior to beginning this journey, and those do not fade away or become less of a priority because you took on this program. You know from how life works that commitments are going to arise that were not planned for whatsoever. Luckily, you have already given yourself the solutions.

You did this and it is not a small thing. Just as you shouldn't compare your workouts to anyone else's, forming, keeping, and adjusting the type of schedule you have is an accomplishment that cannot be taken from you. You didn't back down from that challenge. Instead, you made lasting changes that incorporated the routines instead of just adding them. You already know how to best do this to suit your lifestyle! You have already created the guideline with your original method of scheduling!

It sounds simplistic, but it really is the best approach. Scheduling conflicts *will occur* because life didn't stop, but your ability to be flexible in the face of that didn't stop either. Seeing your workouts as important and deserving priority will give a more balanced perspective. Most of the time, when schedule conflicts derails a program, it is because almost everything that came up immediately became more important than your commitment to working out. By adjusting that mindset, you will find yourself more prepared and rarely caught off guard.

Overexertion

Another common and quite broad subject that may occur during this journey is overexerting yourself. This can take many forms, but it usually leads to injury and eventually becomes a complete disruption to the process. You will certainly be asked to push yourself during the routines, but the absolute rule is that there is a massive difference between the burn of a good muscle stretch and a painful movement. The key, as discussed before, is moderation.

There may be times when you feel that you are not being challenged and you need to add onto the routine. This is a very normal occurrence, and there is a guide in each section of the program to adding sets or reps to your session. Not only is this common, but it is recommended if you are not getting enough of that routine. You should feel challenged and pushed throughout the program, but your safety and health should be foremost in your mind.

This is where your time away from the workout environment is still linked directly to the program. Everything from your sleep patterns, sleeping positions, posture, times spent looking at screens, to the endless other person reasons will have a correlation to your growth and success. You wouldn't be able to conduct the workout and then begin to drink heavily and slouch in front of a TV for six hours the moment you leave. That is an extreme example, but the premise remains true—the way you act in your life is an extension of the way you workout, and vice versa. The two are not possible to separate and they really shouldn't be separate.

There is a danger in creating too much of a barrier between your workout routine and the remainder of your life. A jarring transition will occur every time you go from life to working out and then back. The difference would be so drastic that you run a high risk of developing anxiety about exercising or of having problems applying the lessons of the program to anything outside the workout area.

There are two ways to help avoid injury and still challenge yourself the correct way: resting correctly, and knowing how to increase impact during a session.

Your schedule has Rest Days to ensure your body recovers, but just as important is your resting time between sets. You have been taking breaks to breathe or hydrate in between your sets, but are you doing it the right way? Depending on the type of exercise, you'll need to rest differently as well:

- After running you should hydrate and rest for between 2-4 minutes. Avoid resting too long before the next exercise.
- To help build endurance you lower the rest periods to 30-60 seconds. Do this sparingly as it is an easy way to cause injury or cramping.
- Maintain focus during your rests. Control your breathing and avoid staying stationary.

Once you have ensured your rest periods are being used

correctly, the next step is learning the proper method to add to an exercise to increase the impact and challenge.

One way to increase a set's impact is to include a *Power Set*.

A Power Set has no specific amount of reps, instead it finishes when you have reached a limit. For example, if you are doing push ups and following a 5-rep, 3-set session, you will begin a fourth set and continue doing push ups until you cannot maintain correct form. As always, notice the difference between reaching that limit and pushing yourself past a healthy point! You can sporadically add Power Sets to your routine, but avoid overexerting and causing an avoidable injury.

Then there is the option of creating a *Superset*. A Superset is made when a series of workouts focus on the same muscle area and has similar forms. Remove the rest periods in-between the sets and instead make a fluid transition from one exercise into the other. Doing this creates more isolation on a muscle group and causes more fatigue, leading to hypertrophy and the opportunity to build those specific muscles.

If this is your desired option, you must take into account that your rest period following a Superset is a particular event. Do not make a sudden stop; instead, ease into the rest by staying in motion. Control your breathing and avoid sitting or remaining motionless.

A third option if you are looking to add to a set is a Cluster Set. This is only to be used if the entire workout, all reps and sets within, are minimally challenging. Once you complete the sets in an exercise, take a full rest period and then repeat the entire exercise again. This doesn't give the intensity or impact of the previous options, but increases the strength training within the workout.

A Cluster Set is a rare choice and needs to be observed carefully. Note in your journal how you feel after the first time you complete a Cluster Set directly after, later that day, and the next day. You must ensure that there is no negative fallout. Your health is the ultimate goal!

Boredom

Six months is not a small length of time, and your commitment to it is commendable! That being said, when dealing with that extent of time, you encounter the possibility that boredom occurs. Do not be disheartened or stray from that place of no judgement. That perspective got you to this point, and it is going to keep you going! A basic but effective key to remember right away is to put away the massive, overhanging stigma related to boredom. Especially in regards to a workout routine, the idea of boredom can be catastrophic. It has most likely signalled the beginning of the end in some of the past attempts you had, so it carries that weight forward until the proper actions are taken.

There is a power in recognizing what something truly is and pulling away the curtain. Most fears are as scary as they are because of lingering, attached memories and feelings. This is no different and should be approached the same. The more you learn about a subject, the more power you have over it in regards to changing a perspective. Boredom is in the same class as laziness and tends to function in the same way as well. The fear of laziness tends to bring on anxiety as well. That usually leads to overthinking the problem which, over time, will cause the image and impact of that fear to magnify exponentially! Before you know it, time has passed and you actually fell into the trap of laziness while still being afraid of being lazy.

When you fear boredom and your thought process becomes focused on making sure you aren't bored, you create a fast-paced, uninterested theme. The retention of interest wanes quicker and the desire to do something becomes a lack of action in anything. The cycle of boredom restarts and the rut continues. Instead, confront it directly. You will still feel that initial fear at first, but the more times you recognize the pattern and identify the trigger, you have already removed much of the power. By taking action on that trigger, you take further steps. With a positive spin now, before you know it you have conquered that moment, moved past it, and are ready to continue in growth.

This program is designed to not only provide physical growth, but also mental stimulation. Every month provides a wide variety of workouts that also vary from one session to the next. Despite this consistent variety, there is a good chance that you will feel a sense of monotony at some point in this process. Do not try and simply ignore those feelings of boredom; that solves nothing and will allow it to fester until it becomes a complete lack of motivation. Instead, confront it directly as you have done with road bumps and pitfalls along the way!

Don't be afraid to note when you get a wave of that boredom. Instead, see if you can pinpoint what brought it on. Perhaps a certain exercise tends to drag for you and takes you out of the moment, or you notice that certain days tend to drain you and create a sense of exhaustion that carries into the next workout or, worse, carries into your personal life.

Another option you shouldn't shy away from is changing up your atmosphere. Maybe adding music on certain days or only for specific workouts would add a motivational theme to a difficult day? These are the types of questions you must explore as you combat monotony. Honesty and accountability with yourself has been foundational in getting you here, so trust that and trust yourself to make positive changes when these unmotivated moments hit.

As you make your way through the program and you encounter any of these problem areas we discussed, you should feel empowered to handle them! Recognizing patterns and confronting them will result in huge positive changes! You are worth that effort and you have given yourself so much strength that will carry forward long after you complete the workouts.

Celebrate that and yourself!

The basics of troubleshooting really comes down to understanding the possible problems. Knowledge is power, and the goal is to empower yourself with as much preparedness as possible! While a large amount of information was covered there is a beauty in simplicity—you have all the ability! In breaking down each problem rather than letting it overwhelm you, the solution presents itself and also gives you a guide for future problems.

Even if you find an issue arises that wasn't specifically covered, you are sure to navigate those unsure times by simply utilizing the tools you've already learned! Be honest with yourself about the problem, review your notes or think of a time when you encountered a similar issue, and finally find a way to positively repair the situation.

Chapter Summary

- Are you approaching this chapter from a place free of judgement?
- What distractions have you encountered so far?

- Have you taken steps to alter those moments?
- If there are still areas of distraction, make a list that you can refer to as a chapter progresses
- Which problem area relates to you the most?
- Scheduling?
- Overexertion?
- Boredom?
- Are you giving the proper focus to your Rest Days?
- Are you giving your rest periods between sets the same focus?
- Have you familiarized yourself with the three options for adding intensity and impact to a workout?
- Power Set?
- Superset?
- Cluster Set?
- Have you been feeling bored or have a sense of monotony?
- If so, have you taken steps to recognize what brings it on or is causing it to linger?

CHAPTER EIGHT: THE COOL DOWN

Throughout this entire experience, there has been one absolute that you should walk away with: positivity!

The amount of effort and time put into this program is an exemplary accomplishment and you deserved those positive changes! I know there have been times when even the most meticulously planned schedule hits speed bumps and gets disrupted, and yet you pushed forward!

You've been honest with yourself since the first day and you deserve the same honesty in return: a great deal was asked of you. That is the simple truth. Changes are never easy and you did it while applying important life lessons along the way. At no point should this be a small event in your mind; it is worth joy and celebration!

You were asked to alter your diet, adjust your sleep patterns, push yourself physically, fine-tune yourself mentally, and all the while maintaining a space free from judgement. Perhaps while you were in the midst of the journey, you didn't see the list of goals you were checking off; but having them laid out in front of you now should elicit pride!

Actually, take a moment, as we have many times before, and think of those moments that you weren't sure you were going to continue. I know there were days where time dragged, where an exercise felt like a bored motion, and still you persevered! By going back in your mind, you will get a better view of all the times you overcame! Little by little, you built yourself up and trusted the tools we gave you to find success.

Now it is up to you! There is no reason why you should stop now! You've created a new, healthy, positive lifestyle and that is worth hanging on to. You've used ingenuity to customize in many areas that were presented to you, and there is no doubt you will maintain from here on out!

Create your own routines and process to make sure this change is one of permanence. You have all the capability in the world, and you have proved it time and time again! You've gotten very good at taking the time to review your Journal and recognize patterns, so now you can keep putting that into action!

Whatever methods you determine will work best to help you keep this change in your life, move forward in it with the same lack of judgement you used and have grown within. Your honesty served you well and gave you a better understanding of what works and does not work in different aspects of your life. These accomplishments are no small feat and will continue to prove invaluable!

Again, congratulations, because you have truly bettered yourself! Let's take this last time to celebrate together and recognize your milestone! You are strong and you are better than when you started, and that is certainly something!

FINAL WORDS

This has been quite the journey!

During this process, a bond developed that created the trust between the reader and the program! This is not by accident, and your success was the goal of every action you took!

If this was the sort of journey you would want to explore more of, then there is a community ready to help!

The Daily Jay group on Facebook is a group of experts in their fields working together to provide the most immersive, life-impacting workouts that are possible! With a wide range of subjects at the ready and tips for a continued betterment of your life, this is a safe space for discovering more in this new world of positive health.

Our page and community are not only focused on Calisthenics, but anything fitness and health related! A wide range of subjects and people to help with all your questions, or if you simply want to learn!

If this was an experience that bettered you, which I am sure it did considering all the effort you put forth, then please stop by and see if we can help you!

ACKNOWLEDGMENTS

Image Credit: Shutterstock.com

www.ingramcontent.com/pod-product-compliance
Lightning Source LLC
Chambersburg PA
CBHW072205100526
44589CB00015B/2368